The Extension Activities Handbook

(A Guide to Scouting with the Handicapped)

The Scout Association
25 Buckingham Palace Road,
London, SW1W 0PY.

The Extension Activities Handbook

(A Guide to Scouting with the Handicapped)

Editor
David Harwood

Illustration
Peter Harrison

Design
David Goodman

SBN 85165 030 9

First Edition/First Printing
September 1972.

Second Printing
May 1973

Printed in Great Britain by
**Kent Paper Company Ltd.,
London and Ashford, Kent.**

Contents

Foreword

by **Leonard Robinson,**

Headquarters Commissioner for Extension Activities, 1962 to 1971 (now Chairman World Extension Scouting Committee).

No longer is a boy or young man described as a handicapped Scout. He might be called a Scout with a handicap, but in essence he is a *Scout*. This is not playing with words but is the most important point of the policy of The Scout Association in this respect that a boy becomes a *Scout* when he understands the Scout Law and makes the Scout Promise.
It is hoped that this book will be widely read, not only by those who already have, or who are actively considering having, boys with handicaps in their Groups, but by *all* Scouters in *all* Sections in *every* Group. This book is neither a learned treatise on, nor a medical manual about the treatment of boys with handicaps. It is a book about Scouting. It has been written by someone who had little experience of people with handicaps. He set about the task by asking the kind of questions a Scouter might ask, searching for information and enlisting the help of experts from within and outside the Scout Movement. The result is this practical, factual and concise guide to Scouting with the handicapped. It contains the essential information a Scouter wants and needs to know about Scouting with the handicapped and details of how to set about doing it.
I commend this book in the knowledge that with the understanding that you will derive from its pages, you will give boys who are handicapped a real sense of belonging.

December 1971.

CHAPTER 1

No one is Perfect

The Boys

How many times have you been amazed, pleased surprised or disappointed by the boys and young men in the Cub Scout Pack, the Scout Troop or the Venture Scout Unit with which you work? Probably on every occasion you meet them. Each boy is an individual with his own personality and his own capabilities. No two boys are alike. Your Section is a kaleidoscope of individuals which, like a kaleidoscope, changes its patterns as younger ones join and the older members move up into the next Section. You come to know each member as an individual, and to understand his physical and intellectual strengths and weaknesses, his likes and dislikes. You give him extra instruction and encouragement when he finds a requirement difficult. You insist on a high standard in those areas of activity where you know he has ability, and you expect him to do his best in others. What this amounts to is recognising that not one of the boys or young men in your section is perfect.

You

Can you meet all the requirements of every part of the training programme (including the proficiency badges) of the Section in which you are a Scouter? Your answer must be 'No', because in some instances you do not have the *knowledge*, and/or the *qualifications* and in others you lack the physical or technical skills. If you disagree with this statement, look again at the relevant pages of *Policy, Organisation and Rules – Part Four, Training Badges and Awards.* In a word this can be described as INABILITY (but *not* inefficiency or incompetence).

Do you always take part in and enjoy every aspect of your Section's programme? Again, the answer is probably 'No', for one or more of three main reasons.

1. FEAR – the sight of blood may make you feel queasy, you may not have a head for heights; you may be afraid of flying.

2. PERSONAL DISLIKE – there must be some things which you do not like doing. Sometimes you may have to get on and do them because they are essential, but on other occasions you have a choice, and presumably you select those which you like doing best.
3. MEDICAL – you may have a medical condition which prevents you from fully participating in certain activities either permanently (e.g. hay fever or a heart disease) or temporarily (e.g. influenza or a broken leg).

Inabilities, fears, personal dislikes and medical conditions are present in every individual because, quite simply, no one is perfect.

To admit you are inadequate in some respects is neither a sign of weakness, nor something of which to be ashamed, providing (1) you *try* to overcome your inadequacies within the limits of your intellectual and physical powers; (2) you *accept* that there are many things you will never know and cannot hope to achieve; (3) you *do* what you can do to the best of your ability; (4) you *obtain* help from others (who will have their limitations, too) who have the skills, knowledge or ability to do those things which you cannot do. And if you have made the Scout Promise (which you must have done) you will have already accepted these provisos. All this is plain common sense, and what applies to you applies to the boys or young men whom you lead as well.

Integration

Since no-one is perfect it follows that everyone has a number of intellectual and physical handicaps, though some people, through no fault of their own, have handicaps which are more obvious or pronounced than others. Some are born with a handicap: they can never experience a so-called normal life. Others contract a disease or are involved in an accident which restricts the scope of some of the activities in which they previously participated: they have to re-adjust their lives to their more limited capabilities. However, in most cases, they not only ask to be accepted purely and simply as a person, but also nature often develops in them some other faculty to an astonishing extent. It is, perhaps, nature's way of partially compensating the individual. But this compensation has value only if they have (i) the guts to use it . . . and they usually do, and (ii) the opportunity to use it . . . and too often this is denied to them outside the spheres of education and the activities of the specialist Societies and Organisations. It is in their leisure time activities that Scouting can remove many of the barriers (most of which are artificial and

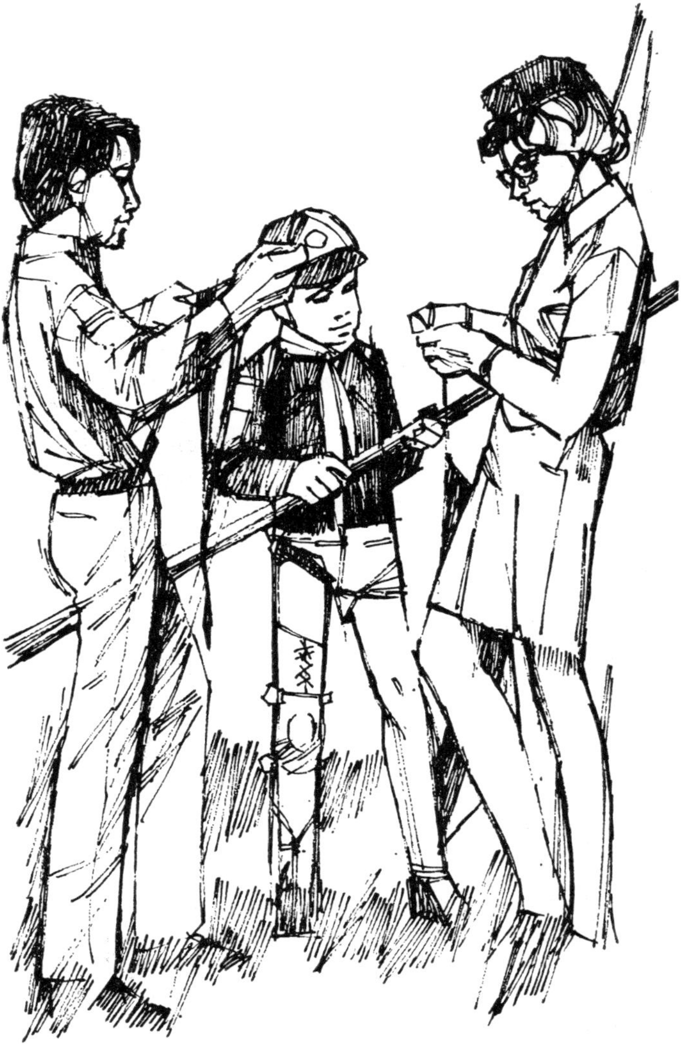

unreasonable) which still divide the handicapped from the ordinary members of society. Much has, and is, being done, but there's a lot more which could be done.

Some Definitions

HANDICAP: 'Physical, emotional, academic or any other incapability which puts a person at a disadvantage compared with his fellows.'

DISABILITY: 'A condition which prevents a person doing something . . . physical incapacity caused by injury or disease.'

NORMAL: 'Conforming to standard, regular, usual, typical.'

EXTEND: Has a number of definitions. In the context of this book it means: 'To reach out to encompass and include.'

A Distinction

In fairness to all, particularly to the individual boy or young man, a different *method of approach* to Scouting (but NOT a different kind of Scouting) is necessary with some forms of handicap, particularly the educationally sub-normal and those with certain other intellectual or social handicaps. Just as physical handicaps are classified into various types, so are intellectual handicaps: the latter cannot and must not be 'lumped together' into one all-embracing category. Chapters 3 and 4 give practical information about various types of handicap and Chapter 8 outlines the policy and practice of Scouting in Extension Groups for those with handicaps. Two points need to be clearly stated here.

1. While every opportunity is taken of integrating a boy with a handicap into an ordinary Group, for some boys Scouting on a week-by-week basis can be more successful and enjoyable in an Extension Group. They would be quite out of their depth in an ordinary Group. This does *not,* however, mean isolating them from the wider aspects and activities of Scouting.

2. The only requirement for a boy to become a *Scout* is that he should make the Promise and understand the Law. Cub Scouts must understand the Cub Scout Law and make the Cub Scout Promise, and Scouts must understand the Scout Law and make the Scout Promise. A boy cannot become a member of the Movement unless he has an understanding of the Promise and the Law, no matter how simple that understanding may be.

CHAPTER 2

The Background

A Reminder

'The Aim of The Scout Association is to encourage the physical, mental and spiritual development of young people so that they may take a constructive place in society. The Method of achieving the Aim of the Association is by providing an enjoyable and attractive scheme of progressive training, based on the Scout Promise and Law and guided by adult leadership.'

Scouting recognises that any organisation which adopts an exclusively insular and introspective attitude is doomed to eventual self-destruction. To develop, expand and thrive, an organisation needs to advance with the times without compromising its principles, and to undergo constant and consistent evolution without losing its identity, its objectives and its close contact with its membership.

Scouting with the handicapped needs to be in accord with current educational and medical policy and practice. If not, it will fall foul of those who are responsible for a much larger and, to be realistic, more important part of an individual boy's life – his education and medical care – and, in so doing, is likely to *prevent* those boys from becoming *Scouts*. No parent, teacher or doctor is going to encourage a child to join an organisation which is literally going to do him more harm than good.

The History

When the 'Disabled Scouts' Branch was formed in the United Kingdom in 1926, some boys with handicaps were already active in Scouting. Two years later the title of the Branch was changed to 'Special Tests', and in 1936 it became known as the Handicapped Scout Branch. At that time it was the general practice to segregate those with handicaps from the rest of the community. Scouting met the challenge and Groups were formed in hospitals and special schools.

Since that time countless boys and young men with handicaps have proved conclusively by what they have done that Scouting has offered them challenge, opportunity and achievement, and, conversely, that Scouting has learnt much, and has much to learn from them.

The principles of care, treatment and attitudes to those with handicaps have changed radically in the past few decades. Medical opinion favours the child with a handicap being allowed to lead as normal a life as possible, i.e. 'integration' rather than 'segregation'. Educationally, the tendency is to look at the functional handling of children rather than their 'types' of handicap. The rapid and encouraging advances of medical science and technology have in some cases eradicated diseases, in others it has brought new hope to those for whom only recently there was no hope. There are still many intellectual and physical conditions whose cause and cure are, as yet, unknown. Sometimes progress in one sphere unfortunately has unpredicted side-effects in another, creating new problems. Medical research has also discovered conditions which previously went undetected or were not fully understood.

It was in the light of these developments that in 1967 the name 'Handicapped Scout Branch' was changed to Extension Activities, and the scope extended to include the boy with a handicap into the field of ordinary Scouting. This was no 'revolutionary' change, but rather a speeding up of the 'evolution' which had been going on, enabling a more efficient organisation to be established and a more enlightened approach to be made to Scouting with boys who are handicapped.

However, many children with handicaps continue to be educated in special day or residential schools which have specialist teachers, ancilliary staff and facilities. In a number of these schools there are long-established Scout Groups led by Scouters who have the aptitude and experience for leading these boys. (See Scouting in Special Schools, page 70).

The Opportunity and the Challenge

'One aspect of how Scouting helps children with handicaps is to prepare them for integration into a predominantly non-handicapped community by receiving the child into an ordinary Group as an individual – *not* as a category. For a child with a handicap the opportunity of finding his own limits and potentialities is of great importance in developing the shell he must create for his protection as he grows up. Physical and mental hurts come to us all and it is happiest when the small ones come early.' – *Countess Estelle Bernadotte of Wisborg, Sweden.*

CHAPTER 3

The Organisation

National

The governing body of The Scout Association in the United Kingdom is the Committee of the Council. There are three principal Sub-Committees of the Committee of the Council – General Purposes, Finance, and Programme and Training. Each Sub-Committee is responsible for a number of Boards. The *National Extension Activities Board* comes under the auspices of the Programme and Training Sub-Committee, with the Headquarters Commissioner for Extension Activities as its Chairman, and a member of the Headquarters staff from the Programme and Training Department as its Secretary. The Board's membership is drawn from inside and outside the Scout Movement, and includes specialists in education, medicine and social welfare. The Board meets at least twice a year and its work includes:

1. Advising the Movement on training and activities for boys with handicaps.
2. Keeping abreast of medical thought and practice to enable the Movement to keep up-to-date in its methods and techniques.
3. Developing activities for boys with handicaps.
4. Acting as the liaison body between Headquarters, the Movement, and with specialists and organisations concerned in the training and education of children with handicaps.

County

Each Scout County has – or should have – an Assistant County Commissioner (Extension Activities) or a County Extension Adviser. He or she is a member of the County team and of the County Programme and Training Sub-Committee. His functions are:

1. To advise the County Commissioner and the County Team on the development of Extension Activities in the County.
2. To maintain liaison with Headquarters.
3. To advise and maintain liaison with District Commissioners in the County.

4. To find and train suitable District Extension Advisers, after consulting the District Commissioners.
5. To advise and maintain liaison with District Extension Advisers and to support the systematic extension of the work among handicapped boys who are not in Scouting.
6. To maintain liaison with Educational, Medical and Social Welfare Authorities.

District

A District Extension Adviser is a member of the District Team. He or she is a member of the Programme and Training Sub-Committee. The appointment of a District Extension Adviser depends upon the potential for Extension Activities in the District, and sometimes an Adviser will be responsible for more than one District. The Adviser's work covers similar fields to the County Adviser, but at District level. In addition, his or her functions are:

1. Liaison with the District Commissioner and Assistant District Commissioners.
2. Knowledge of all the Groups and their Leaders in the District.
3. The integration of young people with a handicap into Scout Groups which do not specialise in dealing with Scouts with a handicap.

Group

The principal purpose of those concerned with Extension Activities at District, County and National levels is to be of help and assistance to the Scouters in the Groups. They are there to be used. Their expertise, knowledge and advice should not only be sought, but should also enable those in ordinary Groups to more easily absorb boys with handicaps into their Sections.

The most important person is the boy. When the Leaders or the *Scouts* in an ordinary Group are considering having a boy with a handicap in their Pack, Troop or Unit, questions naturally arise, such as 'What is the nature of the handicap? How does it affect him? To what extent will his handicap affect *his* Scouting and that of the boys who are already Cub Scouts, Scouts or Venture Scouts? Will we need any special facilities or equipment, etc?'

In the next chapter you will find some of the answers in layman's language and in note form. It is intended to be a *guide* to enable you to decide whether or not your Section or Group can take a particular boy.

CHAPTER 4

Physical Handicaps

Introduction

Although the Department of Education and Science has an official list of handicapping conditions, the categories are primarily medical and educational. They give little guidance to a young person's capacity for taking part in activities outside school or in adult life. Much will depend upon the individual's personality, intelligence, the support he receives from parents and/or others and the extent to which education or therapy has been successful in minimising the effects of the handicap or in developing his skills and general resourcefulness.

More often than not handicaps cannot be seen in distinct black and white terms but rather in varying shades of grey. There is a great danger in attempting to hang a label round an individual's neck. This approach is not only inhuman but also can do irreparable harm to the individual. There is also the very important point that some individuals have more than one handicap. It is not always wise to try and place them in a particular category as each person reacts differently to his handicap. Each person must be considered as an individual. The notes under each heading which follow give factual information about various handicaps.

Blindness and Partial Sight

What It Is:

BLINDNESS: those who have no sight or whose sight is, or likely to become, so defective that they require education by methods not involving the use of sight.

THE PARTIALLY SIGHTED: those who, by reason of defective vision, cannot follow the normal regime of ordinary schools without detriment to their sight or to their educational development, but can be educated by special methods involving the use of sight.

How it affects young people:

It will affect their mobility, orientation and (to a lesser degree) their social integration.

Education:
Most blind children are educated in special boarding schools and Extension Groups may be formed for them at the school. A proportion of those with partial sight are educated in special boarding schools but the majority attend special day schools and can therefore join ordinary Scout Groups.

Safety and Welfare

Advisable additional facilities:
None.

Points to watch during meetings, activities, etc.:
(a) Stability of furniture indoors and ensure items are always in the same place. Give prior warning of equipment put in unusual places and check that doors are not left ajar, etc. Take particular care to carefully store such potentially dangerous items as axes and saws.

(b) On outdoor activities give detailed description of obstacles and immediate landmarks, e.g. there is nothing worse than falling over a bicycle left in the wrong place.

(c) Encourage everyone to describe what is going on and avoid silences or sudden noises. Speak normally. The tone of voice is important because it expresses the speaker's feelings, which the blind cannot see from *facial* expressions.

Routine First Aid treatment required:
None.

Additional Items for First Aid Kit:
None.

Knowledge of Aids and Equipment:
The catalogue of equipment especially provided for the blind by the Royal National Institute for the Blind is essential.

Programme

Activities in which a boy can most likely participate:
Those not requiring the use of sight. It is an advantage if the remaining senses (touch, smell, taste and hearing) are used to a greater degree.

Activities in which the boy can least likely participate:
Any solely visual activities. The partially sighted cannot benefit from demonstrations and visual aids and, if totally blind, will not be able to read instructions unless presented in Braille.

Useful training and teaching techniques:
(a) Training methods are generally facilitated by tactile (i.e.

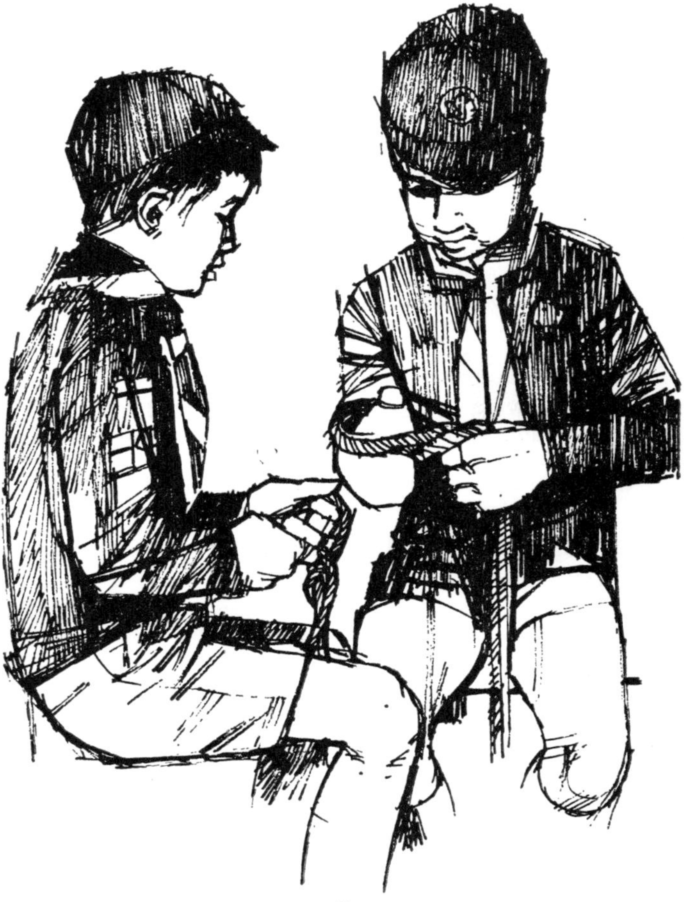

connected with the sense of touch) aids. Give the boy time to learn about his environment, particularly if the activity involves movement over a large area. If being taught at a table or bench, let him feel the layout and placing of equipment. Let him handle the tools to be used, as you are naming them, describing their use and emphasising special ways of handling to ensure safety. Once the boy has gained this impression, avoid confusing him by unnecessary movement of furniture, equipment and tools.

(b) If instructing an otherwise sighted group, ensure that the boy is near enough to hear clearly or, if partially sighted, to see as much as he is able; check, therefore, that there is plenty of light. When demonstrating to others, have a duplicate set of equipment for the blind boy to handle, his movements being guided by another instructor. Allow the blind or partially sighted to demonstrate to the other boys what they might have to do in the dark, e.g. house on fire at night, broken torch on a night hike, etc.

(c) A basic knowledge of Braille would be helpful.

Additional games and activities equipment:

There are embossed maps, Braille compasses, etc., available and *The Scout Handbook* is published in Braille. *The Cub Scout Handbook* has been recorded. A tape recorder will be a great asset. Most other equipment can be easily adapted.

Reference Material

The Royal National Institute for the Blind (address page 93) have a large number of useful and informative pamphlets and leaflets.

The Guide Dogs for the Blind Association (address page 93)

Deafness and Partial Hearing

What it is:

THE DEAF: those with impaired hearing who require education by methods suitable for pupils with little or no naturally acquired speech or language.

THE PARTIALLY HEARING: those with impaired hearing whose development of speech and language, even if retarded, is following a normal pattern and who require for their education special arrangements or facilities though not necessarily all the educational methods used for deaf pupils.

A person who is born deaf or becomes deaf before acquiring speech patterns loses the basic essentials of language and communication. A person who becomes deaf later in life loses the ease and spontaneity of communication.

How it affects young people:

Loneliness. Difficulty in communication and, if totally deaf, much of life's experience could pass by. Adolescence is a particularly difficult time when allied to deafness. Deaf young people will have a smaller vocabulary than those with unimpaired hearing – they should *never* be referred to as deaf and dumb.

Education:

Traditionally (and from geographical necessity in the past) most deaf and partially hearing children go to special boarding schools. Special day schools are more common now and there are many partially hearing units in ordinary schools.

Safety and Welfare

Advisable additional facilities:

None.

Points to watch during meetings, activities, etc.:

(a) Ensure that the deaf boy knows of any danger spots, particularly while camping, potholing, swimming, etc. What would normally be conveyed in conversation could be lost on a deaf boy even if he was wearing an aid. He must have had clear, safe, concise *personal* information. It should never be assumed that the boy knows.

(b) Never blindfold him.

Routine First Aid treatment required:

None.

Additional Items for First Aid Kit:

None.

Knowledge of Aids and Equipment:

The care and use of hearing aids for those who are partially hearing would be helpful.

Programme

Activities in which a boy can most likely participate:

Those which are practical and visual.

Activities in which a boy can least likely participate:

Those which involve complicated verbal explanation beforehand or which demand instant verbal response.

The totally deaf will not benefit from verbal instruction unless they can lip read and the partially deaf, although often helped by hearing aids, often misconstrue what has been said, particularly if there are confusing background noises.

Useful training and teaching techniques:

(a) The oral system of teaching, which involves lip reading, has largely superseded the use of the manual alphabet and sign language at school. Young people who are being taught orally should be encouraged to converse by this method, thus supporting the work of their teachers.

(b) Visual aids are most important for the deaf and audio visual aids for the partially hearing.

(c) Position the boy so that he has a clear, full face view of the instructor. He can then see what is going on and, if able to lip read, is in the best position to understand what is being said. The instructor should face the light and the activity demonstrated should be clearly visible without the clutter of extra unnecessary equipment around it.

(d) Where the boy has to view the demonstration from the same angle as the instructor, verbal instruction may have to be dispensed with while the demonstration is going on, but visual aids such as flannel boards or flip charts may be used to augment the teaching for the whole group, thus drawing less undue attention to the deaf boy.

(e) A deaf boy will miss 'asides' and these are often about precautions or extra 'tips' which makes the job easier. Care should be taken to see that he is not at a disadvantage in this respect.

(f) Expression by tone of voice will be lost.

(g) Expression by facial characteristics assume greater importance and care is needed (e.g. frowning when pulling a boy's leg could be misconstrued by a deaf boy as an indication of disapproval).

Additional games and activities equipment:

A useful item would be amplification equipment and, if there are boys using suitable hearing aids, the Headquarters could be fitted with an inexpensive 'Loop' system, full details of which are in the Royal National Institute for the Deaf booklet *Special Aids to Hearing.*

Reference Material

The Royal National Institute for the Deaf (address page 92) publish an extensive range of booklets and pamphlets. The R.N.I.D. has its own library and an illustrated leaflet describing the library and its various facilities is available from The Chief Librarian/Information Officer. A list of books on hearing and speech, which has been specially prepared for anyone who has had little or no previous knowledge on the problems of hearing and speech is particularly helpful.

The National Deaf Children's Society (address page 92),

which is mainly a parents' organisation, actively co-operates with The Scout Association and all their literature is available free to Scout Groups. Their quarterly magazine *Talk* is distributed free to all who are interested in deaf children.

Epilepsy

What it is:

The term covers a wide variety of disturbances in consciousness ranging from brief interruptions in thought or behaviour to severe fits with convulsions. The two main types of epilepsy are:

(1) Major fits, sometimes known as grand mal.
These can be frightening, especially for anyone seeing them for the first time.
The person will suddenly fall, some without any warning, becoming unconscious and making involuntary convulsive movements which are sometimes violent. Some epileptics have a 'warning' of impending attack and prepare themselves by seeking help, e.g. safety precautions by lying down. There may be a cry or strange noises. There may also be a slight frothing or bubbling at the mouth, occasionally coloured with blood as a result of biting the tongue or lips.
When the attack is over the patient may appear confused or tired for some time.

(2) Minor fits, generally called petit mal.
You may hardly notice these when they occur. They may look like day-dreaming or momentary blankness. Sometimes there is excessive eye-blinking. These short spells of unconsciousness last for only a few seconds. It is very rare for the patient to fall or to show other signs that anything unusual has happened.

(3) There is another type of epilepsy which you may come across (known medically as Psychomotor). It usually consists of repeated involuntary movements associated with a clouding of consciousness. There may be twitching, jerking of plucking movements and these may spread down one side of the body. The patient usually appears to be conscious but may not be able to speak or respond during the attack.
Strictly speaking epilepsy is not cured but in many cases the attacks can be completely controlled and in others they can be greatly reduced in number. Children may grow out of them and even in adult life seizures may cease spontaneously. Usually drugs are employed to control seizures and it is essential that they be taken regularly as prescribed by the physician.

How it affects young people:

The outward signs have been described above. The condition is unpredictable, as also is its effect on other people. It is as well to remember that the boy is unconscious during a fit and is quite unaware of what is going on. Fear, horror, etc., in others becomes immediately apparent to him on recovery. Understanding and acceptance are, therefore, vitally important to the boy's well-being.

Education:

About 90% of young people with epilepsy attend ordinary schools. Severe cases, often associated with other handicaps or mental retardation, may attend special residential schools for epilepsy or special day schools.

Safety and Welfare

Advisable additional facilities:

None. It is advisable for doors, including toilet doors, not to be locked.

Points to watch during meetings, activities, etc.:

(a) All work with fires, axes, etc., should be done under close supervision.

(b) Activities at heights should be avoided. Swimming should *only* be undertaken with the agreement of the boy's parents and doctor and then only under strict and close supervision. He should not be allowed in lonely or inaccessible places unless accompanied.

(c) For camps and outings.
He should have with him a supply of his drugs with full instructions as to the dosage, etc. It is essential that the instructions should be followed.

(d) Severe epileptics are usually best accommodated in extension camps where special facilities (e.g. sleeping in marquees, staff coverage, etc.) can be provided.

(e) Do not assume that epileptics have heard what has been said. Not only is their span of concentration often very limited but they may also be suffering petit mal fits which may render what has been said virtually unintelligible to them. One may be aware of these attacks and therefore take care to repeat again and again until they have shown that they have understood. If the attacks pass unnoticed such an eventuality must always be borne in mind and the requisite patience be shown in training.

Routine first aid treatment required:

The first rule is to keep calm. There is nothing you can do to stop an attack once it has begun. Clear the area around the patient so that he does not injure himself but do not restrain him any more than is absolutely necessary. Do not force anything between his teeth or give him anything to drink. It is not usually necessary to call a doctor unless the attack is followed by others without recovery in between.

Additional items for First Aid Kit:

None.

Knowledge of Aids and Equipment:

None.

Programme

Activities in which a boy can most likely participate:

Almost all activities, but note the comments made in 'Points to Watch' above.

Activities in which the boy can least likely participate:

Swimming, climbing, parts of gymnastics.

Useful training and teaching techniques:

None.

Additional games and activities equipment:

None.

Reference Material

The Epilepsy Information Unit of the British Epilepsy Association (address page 93) publishes three useful pamphlets: *Epilepsy – What To Do; Questions and Answers about Epilepsy; A Teacher's Guide on Epilepsy.* The Advice Section of the Epilepsy Information Unit will always be pleased to advise on any particular problem that may arise.

Epilepsy and Fits, a Family Doctor booklet by Dr. Desmond Pond and Dr. Eric Johnson, 30 pages, published by the British Medical Association.

Diabetes

What it is:

This is a deficiency in natural insulin production resulting in failure to burn up the body's production of glucose – resulting in loss of weight – coma and, if untreated, death.

How it affects young people:

It requires treatment by diet and almost invariably by insulin – giving a balance between the starchy (sugar) foods needed to produce energy and the insulin given.

Education:

Virtually all diabetics attend ordinary schools.

Safety and Welfare

Advisable additional facilities:

None

Points to watch during meetings, activities, etc.:

(a) Check with parents whether the child is liable for insulin reactions. Be armed with glucose in liquid or tablet form for emergency treatment if the child becomes faint. If he becomes unconscious, call a doctor.

(b) Before exercise (games, swimming, cycling, etc.) give extra starch in the form of bread or biscuits, i.e. slowly absorbed foods.

(c) Look for injuries. A small blister or cut can be serious. Sugar logged tissues are unhealthy tissues and cannot heal properly and can turn bad and gangrenous when untreated. Wash thoroughly any scratches or bites, and cover.

(d) Watch for special diets when camping or away from home.

Routine First Aid treatment required:

Glucose may need to be given.

Additional items for First Aid Kit:

Glucose. Thick rubber to prevent clenching of teeth.

Knowledge of Aids and Equipment:

The general advice from a doctor well used to caring for young diabetics. Let the boy rely on, and follow, the advice given by the physician-in-charge and his team (e.g. the dietician, etc.)

Programme

Activities in which a boy is most likely to participate:

All.

Activities in which a boy is least likely to participate:

None.

Useful training and teaching techniques:

None.

Additional games and activities equipment:

None.

Reference Material

The British Diabetic Association (address page 93) publishes a number of pamphlets, booklets, etc. Of special interest are: *Introducing Diabetes; Diabetes in Children; Diet and Diabetics; Medical and Social Aspects of Caring for Diabetic Children; The Effects of Exercise on the Young Diabetic; Hypoglycaemia; Swimming for the Diabetic.*

Other publications and lists are available on application to the British Diabetic Association.

Muscular Dystrophy

What it is:

A widespread wasting of the muscles, leading to loss of voluntary movement. It is a progressive disease, which primarily affects boys and runs in families. In its worst and most common form it affects children (who may not survive their 'teens).

How it affects young people:

In time the condition becomes increasingly apparent and the patient is confined to a wheel chair. At first it may look as though a small boy is just slow at walking with a peculiar waddling gait, then he finds walking more difficult and cannot raise his arms. He may be in a wheel chair by nine or ten years of age.

Mental ability is not affected by the disease.

Incontinence is not a problem.

Education:

The young person with muscular dystrophy usually attends an ordinary school for as long as possible, then a special school, either day or residential, according to family circumstances and local facilities.

Safety and Welfare

Advisable educational facilities:

Adapted toilets and ramps for the wheel chair may be necessary if the disease has progressed to this stage *but* these adapted toilets and ramps are not essential. What usually happens is that the boys are wheeled about quite happily by other boys or lifted up the odd step, etc. Convenient transport would be a necessity for bringing the boy to and from meetings and activities.

Points to watch during meetings, activities, etc.:

(a) Children with muscular dystrophy have to be particularly careful not to get chest infections as their muscle power (for coughing, etc.) is weaker than other children. They should therefore be well wrapped up in cold or damp weather. Unless special provision has been made (e.g. at an Extension camp) it is probably wiser for the boy not to go on week-end camping expeditions or to stay overnight anywhere, partly to avoid the risk of chest infection and partly because some of the boys need turning at night to alter their position in bed.

Routine First Aid treatment required:

None.

Additional items for the First Aid Kit:

None.

Knowledge of Aids and Equipment:

The boy himself will be able to explain about his own equipment and special requirements. For example, some may have a strap to hold their chests near the back of their wheel chairs, but not all the boys with muscular dystrophy will need this aid.

Programme

Activities in which the boy is most likely to participate:

Those using hands and brain. Sitting down games (where the boy is in a wheel chair).

Activities in which the boy is least likely to participate:

Running about.

Useful training and teaching techniques:

Nothing special as long as the boy is able to see clearly.

Additional games and activities equipment:

None.

Reference Material

The Muscular Dystrophy Group of Great Britain (address page 93), publishes leaflets about the disease, and gives information which may be useful to sufferers.

Special Note:

Going into Cub Scouts and then into Scouts can be a great help, especially as the boy may still be on his feet and not wheel chair bound at the age of a Cub Scout.

Poliomyelitis

What it is:

Until relatively recently this disease was common in Britain, but now it occurs very rarely. The infection leaves children with varying degrees of paralysis which can affect any of the voluntary muscles of the body. Children may be left with paralysis of the arms, the legs, the trunk or respiratory muscles or, in severe cases, they may be totally paralysed.

How it affects young people:

It depends upon which muscles are affected. Whereas a boy with paralysed arms and legs may need help up steps or

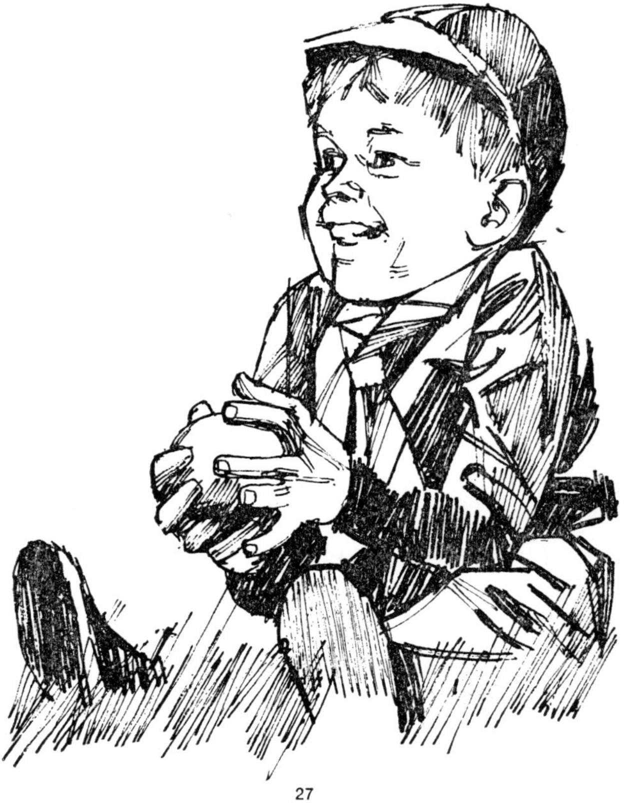

over a stile, those with respiratory paralysis are at particular risk from any colds and coughs that are about and need to be watched carefully.

Education:

Polios usually attend ordinary schools but this will depend on other circumstances (e.g. home conditions, age when afflicted, degree of disability, etc.)

Safety and Welfare

Advisable additional facilities:

Provision of adapted toilets and a ramp for the wheel chair will be required in the more severe cases.

Points to watch during meetings, activities, etc.:

(a) Supervision should be exercised to ensure that the boy does not run undue risk but generally he will wish to disregard his disability.

(b) Activities on which he is engaged should be within his capacity.

(c) A polio is normally a fit person who has a paralysed limb.

Routine First Aid treatment required:

None.

Additional items for the First Aid Kit:

None.

Knowledge of Aids and Equipment:

A polio often may have one or more of the following: calipers, crutches or wheel chair. Some knowledge of their purpose and handling will be needed.

Programme

Activities:

The spheres of activity in which a polio can participate will depend entirely on the extent of his disability. It does not prevent him from swimming.

Useful training and teaching techniques:

None.

Additional games and activities equipment:

Archery and equipment for field events would be useful.

Reference Material

The British Polio Fellowship (address page 93) publishes an Annual Report and a bi-monthly journal (*The Bulletin*) both of which contain information of interest to the polio.

Migraine

What it is:

Migraine is a prostrating headache followed by vomitting, partial blindness or other forms of visual disturbance, e.g. coloured stars and light flashes. Migraine is a very agonising condition and invariably prostrating while the attack lasts. It is in no sense a serious condition and the patients are invariably extremely healthy individuals in all other respects. It is inherited and linked with asthma, hay fever and uticaria. Epilepsy is sometimes connected but this is rare. Excitement, travel and emotional fatigue, bright light and certain foods are the general trigger factors.
Food should be taken regularly and frequently as fasting also contributes in triggering attacks. Sufferers should be taught to relax before the excitement of travel or of events. Emotional stress of any kind is closely involved.

How it affects young people:

Migraine is likely to strike without warning following excitement, travel, fatigue, bright sunlight, high winds and many other factors. The patient appears to be very ill and in very great pain but recovers quickly after rest and sleep.

Education:

Migraine sufferers attend ordinary schools.

Safety and Welfare

Advisable additional facilities:

None.

Points to watch during meetings, activities, etc.:

(a) Visual disturbances, over exertion, excitement.

Routine First Aid treatment required:

Special medication will be provided by the boy's doctor. Do not offer medication of any kind unless prescribed by his doctor. Check with the boy's parents about his medication. Escort the boy home if practicable, otherwise take him to a darkened room for complete rest and isolation from light and noise and, subject to medical advice, apply a vinegar soaked compress to the head. Full recovery generally occurs after a few hours but in some cases it may require a full night's sleep. Do not fuss but do realise that the patient's pain is intense.

Additional items for the First Aid Kit:

Only those advised by parents and/or doctor.

Knowledge of Aids and Equipment:

None.

Programme

Activities in which a boy is most likely to participate:

All activities, only avoiding those involving undue stress, excitement and over exertion.

Activities in which the boy is least likely to participate:

Always check with parents, but generally avoid horseplay and heavy ragging, for these boys are very sensitive. Avoid bright sunlight and high winds.

Useful training and teaching techniques:

Whenever possible teach the boy to relax as much as possible while playing or working and try to avoid over excitement.

Additional games and activities equipment:

None.

Reference Material

Migraine – What It's All About, available free from the Migraine Trust (address page 93).
The British Migraine Association (address page 92).

Cerebral Palsy

What it is:

Cerebral Palsy is a disorder of movement or of posture due to an injury of an immature (growing) brain. Progressive disorders of posture or of movement are excluded as Cerebral Palsy is not a progressive state. The extent of the handicap ranges from as little as 5% to total disability (i.e. from boys who can run 80 metres in 9.7 seconds to those who cannot even turn the pages of a book or wipe their own nose). Incidence of Cerebral Palsy is roughly seven in every 100,000 births a year. Of these: one will die in infancy; two will be feeble minded (Institute care); one will be severely handicapped (home bound); one will be moderately handicapped; on will be very mildly handicapped and hardly need treatment.

There are three main forms of Cerebral Palsy – spasticy, athetosis and ataxia. Sufferers from all three types are commonly called by the general term 'Spastic'.

The spastic child has muscle weakness, disordered movement and often disturbance in growth and development. It may affect both the limbs on one side of the body (hemiplegia), both the lower limbs (paraplegia) or all four limbs (diplegia).

The main feature of the 'athetoid spastic' is the frequent involuntary movements which mask and interfere with the normal movements of the whole body.

The spastic child with ataxia has an unsteady gait and difficulty in balancing.

Seriously handicapped spastics may have a combination of more than one of these basic categories.

Do not be misled by their looks. Few are mentally deficient, and many are normally as intelligent as those without any handicap at all. Those who are facially deformed are often the most intelligent. So, if they grimace when they speak do not treat them as imbeciles. Some may often be unable to express themselves coherently and others may be unable to co-ordinate voluntary movements or even both.

How it affects young people:

Immaturity, under-developed personality, intolerance, self-centredness due to an early environment (e.g. hospitalisation, total care, etc.), inability to understand at times (lack of early experience). The cerebral palsied seem to have an innate conviction that others must adjust to the cerebral palsied and not the cerebral palsied to others.

Education:

Until recently the cerebral palsied attended special boarding schools. This is now changing. Many go to special day schools or to units attached to ordinary schools and some are accepted in ordinary schools.

Advisable additional facilities:

The less adaptation or additional facility the better. If only one spastic boy is joining a Group it is preferable that no special arrangements be made for him. Special arrangements mean special treatment, means someone special, means someone different. He joins the Group to be just 'one of the boys'.

Points to watch during meetings, activities, etc.:

(a) When helping a boy who is spastic to use his arms or legs, etc., never move fast for if you push or pull a limb it will go into a spasm and your efforts will have been in vain. On the other hand, if any of his muscles are moved slowly the limbs will do what is wanted.

(b) Remember not to agitate the boy for excitement will cause his movements to worsen and the spasm will get worse.

Routine First Aid equipment required:

None.

Additional items for the First Aid Kit:

None.

Knowledge of Aids and Equipment:

See Mechanical Aids (page 64).

Programme

The spheres of activity in which the boy is likely to be able to participate are governed entirely by the degree of the handicap as is the participation of any boy. Leaders will easily decide in which games and activities individual boys can participate and also what additional equipment, if any, is needed.

Reference Material

The Spastics Society (address page 92) publishes a number of useful pamphlets and booklets and a magazine *Spastics News.*

Chest Disease (including Asthma and Cystic Fibrosis)

What it is:

Breathing difficulties, sudden spasms of breathlessness and coughing (asthma) production of phlegm (cystic fibrosis).

How it affects young people:

Asthma – each case has different causes and 'trigger mechanisms' for attacks. They can be psychologically caused by worry, tension, etc., travelling, being away from home or contact with allergens (i.e. substances to which the person is abnormally sensitive, which could be pollen, dust, animal hair, etc.). Asthma may be complicated by bronchitis producing sputum.

Cystic Fibrosis – The boy's chest has a tendency to 'silt up' and anything which could precipitate this must be avoided. This is, however, a rare condition. Care must be taken to avoid coughs and colds.

Education:

It depends entirely on individual circumstances as to whether a young person attends a special boarding school, a special day school or an ordinary school.

Safety and Welfare

Advisable additional facilities:

In cases of allergy, meeting places and programmes must be checked for possible contact with allergens. Cystic fibrotics need privacy and informed assistance for clearing the chest. Travelling distances and conditions must be considered. It is advisable to check with parents and preferably the doctor in each individual case.

Points to watch during meetings, activities etc.:

(a) These boys tend to resent their illness and will try to join in anything that is going on. They must be prevented *very tactfully* from getting over tired or joining in too hectic activities, but they must never be allowed to feel left out or different. Leaders should check with parents and/or doctor for individual points to be watched.

Routine First Aid equipment required:

Chesty boys often have routine breathing exercises to practise. Cystic fibrotics have 'tipping and slapping' routines for chest drainage. Boys may need supervision in the taking of regular medication. Arrangements should be made for local emergency medical aid if the boy is to go outside his home area. Breathing exercises and chest drainage procedures should be learnt.

Additional items for the First Aid Kit:

None.

Knowledge of Aids and Equipment:

None.

Programme

Activities in which the boy is most likely to be able to participate:

Indoor activities including sedentary craftwork. Cystic fibrotics are encouraged to swim and exercise (except where there is a risk of catching cold). Allergic asthmatics need only avoid their own allergens. Leaders should avoid exposing asthmatics to windy conditions: it would be of assistance if the boys had inhalers which they had been taught to use.

Activities in which the boy is least likely to be able to participate:

Camping will present great difficulties (local medical support, avoidance of allergens, supervision of regime, avoidance of over-exertion, etc.) but will be of considerable psychological value if it can be arranged. See Chapter 8. Competitive sports may be ruled out.

Useful training and/or teaching techniques:

None.

Additional games and activities equipment:

Provision of equipment for board games, particularly the more demanding (e.g. chess, halma, mah-jong) may add variety for those debarred from active sports and bored with the usual indoor games.

Reference Material

The Chest and Heart Association (address page 92) publishes books, leaflets and posters, lists of which are available free on request. There is also a list of their Children's Chest Circle Library showing some of the titles recommended to parents. Leaders of Groups containing 'chesty' children or young heart patients would be welcomed as members of the Children's Chest Circle, an organisation principally for the parents of chesty children, which gives advice on general and individual problems, has a postal lending library and a toy library, and publishes a regular newsletter (and a teenage newsletter for the young patients themselves).

The Cystic Fibrosis Research Trust (address page 93) can provide more information about those suffering from this rare disability.

Heart Disease (including Congenital Deformity)

What it is:

Deficiency of heart and circulatory system leading to shortness of breath, blue lips and nails, etc. Boys of Scout age are often in the middle of a series of corrective operations for congenital heart defects.

How it affects young people:

Activities must be carefully rationed and the boy must not over exert himself.

Education:

It depends entirely on the individual circumstances as to whether the young person attends a special boarding school, a special day school or an ordinary school.

Safety and Welfare

Advisable additional facilities:

Transport may be needed in order to conserve the boy's energy for the planned activities. It is advisable to check with the parents and preferably the doctor in each individual case.

Points to watch during meetings, activities, etc.

(a) These boys may resent their illness and will try to join in anything that is going on. They must be prevented *very tactfully* from getting over tired or joining in too hectic activities, but they must never be allowed to feel left out or different. Leaders should check with parents and/or doctor for individual points to be watched. Over-weight children may be on diets.

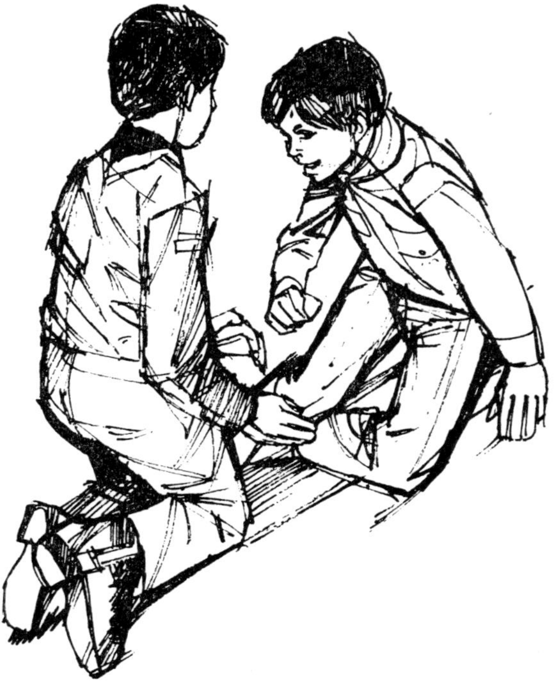

Routine First Aid treatment required:

Boys may need supervision in the taking of regular medications. Arrangements should be made for local emergency medical aid if the boy is to go outside his home area.

Additional items for the First Aid Kit:

None.

Knowledge of Aids or Equipment:

None.

Programme

Activities in which the boy is most likely to be able to participate:

Indoor activities including sedentary craft work.

Spheres of activity in which the boy is least likely to be able to participate:

Camping may present great difficulties (local medical support, supervision of regime, avoidance of over exertion, etc.) but will be of considerable psychological value if it can be arranged. See Extension Camps (pages 73–77). Competitive sports may be ruled out.

Additional games and activities equipment:

Provision of equipment for board games, particularly the more demanding (e.g. chess, halma, mah-jong) may add variety for those debarred from active sports and bored with the usual indoor games.

Reference Material

The Chest and Heart Association (address page 92) publishes books, leaflets and posters, lists of which are available free on request. For details of the Children's Chest Circle, see page 34.

Haemophilia

What it is:

Haemophilia is a blood clotting disorder in which part of the clotting mechanism is defective (i.e. the blood takes longer than normal to clot). This can lead to prolonged bleeding in joints, muscles and soft tissue and severe external cuts often take much longer to heal.

How it affects young people:

Any sudden knocks, strains or twists may set off a bleeding episode which, if left untreated, will cause great pain. If the affected part is a joint, this may become very swollen and stiff, leading to loss of use and possibly to permanent damage.

Education:

Haemophiliacs are educated in all types of school depending on how severely handicapped they are from previous bleeding episodes.

Safety and Welfare

Advisable additional facilities:

None.

Points to watch during meetings, activities, etc.:

(a) Haemophiliacs need to be self-reliant and able to stand up to their particular complaint. They should not be 'wrapped in cotton wool', but rather allowed to join in all activities as far as possible. Most haemophiliacs know their limitations but, boys being boys, they will often try to exceed the limits and the Leader should keep an eye open to try to prevent this. A haemophiliac boy generally knows a great deal about his complaint and can usually be relied on if he says something is wrong. A quiet chat with his parents before he joins the Group would be a good idea and, in addition, it would be sensible to contact the Haemophilia Society which could then supply relevant and useful information and leaflets.

(b) Football, climbing, 'contact' activities, etc., are not suitable and a haemophiliac should be prevented from joining in rough and tumble games.

(c) Any signs of pain or restrictions in movement should be watched for as these could indicate the start of a bleeding episode. It is vitally important that at the *first* sign of such an episode the boy should be taken home or his parents contacted in order that they may arrange for him to receive treatment. If away from home, the boy's haemophilia treatment centre should be contacted (the address of which, with other details, will be on a small card which all haemophiliacs should carry) for advice. If a long way from the boy's normal centre the nearest centre should be contacted. An ordinary hospital is *not sufficient* as it will not have the special drugs needed. The Haemophilia Society will always be pleased to give the address of the nearest centre to wherever the Group is going.

Routine First Aid treatment required:

Ordinary first aid treatment is sufficient for small cuts, etc., but see above for action if the bleeding is more serious.

Additional items for the First Aid Kit:

None.

Knowledge of Aids or Equipment:

Some haemophiliacs use walking sticks or calipers or, from time to time, are confined to wheel chairs but for the majority of the time will be quite mobile (see Mechanical Aids, page 64).

Programme

Spheres of activity in which the boy is most likely to be able to participate:

Sedentary activities requiring no great physical effort, e.g. modelling.

Spheres of activity in which the boy is least likely to be able to participate:

Activities which involve great physical efforts, such as football or running.

Useful training and/or teaching techniques:

None.

Additional equipment for games and activities:

None.

Reference Material

A selection of pamphlets will be supplied to anyone on request to the Haemophilia Society (address page 92).

Spina Bifida and/or Hydrocephalus

What it is:

Spina bifida, which literally means 'split spine', is a condition with which some babies are born. Its causes are not yet known. The spine does not join as it should so the spinal cord is exposed. If it were left like this it is liable to damage and infection so, in most cases now, as soon as possible after birth the baby is operated on to close the spinal column. The most usual trouble spot is the lower part of the back but it may be higher up. Because the spine has not developed normally the nerves have already suffered damage and there is paralysis; this varies from child to child but probably means there is the loss of feeling and malformation of the legs which lead to walking difficulties and often also to lack of control of the bladder and bowels. Their incontinence is nothing to do with 'nerves' nor is it a condition that they can be taught to overcome.

Hydrocephalus – often called 'water on the brain – is fairly often associated with spina bifida though it also occurs independently. Fluid accumulates in the brain abnormally and if untreated this leads to brain damage and because the skull is soft it can be pushed out by pressure and could result in a large head. This condition is now usually treated by putting a valve and tube into the child's head which drains away the excess fluid down into the blood stream.

Education:
The degree of severity varies so much and school placement is an individual matter. A child with these handicaps could thus be educated in a special boarding school, a special day school or an ordinary school but in any event the school will not necessarily be of the same type throughout his school life.

Safety and Welfare

Advisable additional facilities:
Reasonable accessibility to ground floor level, particularly for a wheel chair, and a ground floor lavatory are very desirable and in some cases essential.

Points to watch during meetings, activities, etc.:
(a) The affected limbs of all boys who have some degree of paralysis may be less sensitive to surface feelings. *Guard against them being left near a fire or other source of heat without a guard between them and the fire.* In cold weather make sure that their limbs are kept warm. They are also prone to friction 'burns' on paralysed limbs.

(b) Fractures (often unnoticed for some time) occur in spina bifidas and careful – but unobtrusive – examination of the lower limbs for bruising and swelling is needed.

(c) Attention to their toilet needs is important and on outdoor activities they may have very limited walking capacity or use a wheel chair. Include a plastic urine bottle in your kit and let the boy be assured that you understand his needs and, most important, see to it that you meet them.

(d) At camp, boys may need turning during night.

(e) It is imperative that extra care be taken with these Scouts and that their heads are not accidentally or otherwise knocked. If this does happen then parents or school authorities must be informed of the incident as special care must be taken or medical help may be reqiured. These Scouts are more often than not strapped into their wheel chairs as a safety precaution.

Special Note:
The number of those with spina bifida surviving to Scout age is increasing rapidly following modern surgical techniques and medical treatment. Their leisure time is of great importance as they need greater support having often had fewer opportunities to make friends and to join in group activities due to their handicap, hospitalisation and parental caution.

Routine First Aid Treatment required:
None other than mentioned above.

Additional items for the First Aid Kit:

None in this sense – do not forget the plastic bottle.

Knowledge of Aids and Equipment:

As stated, some spina bifidas *may* use calipers, a wheel chair, etc. A spina bifida may have special medical appliances attached to his body to alleviate incontinence: the application and removal of these appliances require foreknowledge and training.

Programme

A spina bifida or hydrocephalic will fit in with the programme with little adjustment in rather a similar manner as the spastic. Fullest integration is perhaps the most important aim. Depending on the degree of the handicap, physical activities can be undertaken, although games or hikes on foot may be impossible. Opportunities to have experience in cultural activities and such subjects as natural history, collections, etc., should enrich a boy's life, i.e. developing interests where the handicap will not be an obstacle.

Useful training and teaching techniques:

Nothing special.

Additional games and equipment:

Heat shields for protection from fire when cooking.

Reference Material

A number of books, pamphlets and leaflets are published by the Association for Spina Bifida and Hydrocephalus (address page 93).

Brittle Bones (Osteogenesis Imperfecta)

What it is:

A defect from birth of the bony skeleton due to faulty bone production and resulting in brittle bones which may break easily after trivial injuries. It is associated with a peculiar blue colour of the eye balls.

How it affects young people:

Fractures are easily sustained, often during normal activities when some minor accident occurs.

Education:

At an ordinary school.

Safety and Welfare

Advisable additional facilities:

None.

Points to watch during meetings, activities, etc.:

(a) The least snap, the least pull will cause a fracture. Although these boys should not be over protected, they must be treated with care and circumspection and not allowed to play violent games.

Routine First Aid treatment required:

None in this sense, although adults and boys would be wise to ensure they know how to treat fractures.

Additional items for the First Aid Kit:

None in particular, apart from ensuring that there is sufficient for treatment of fractures.

Knowledge of Aids and Equipment:

Some may be wearing leg splints.

Programme

Apart from extra care being exercised in more boisterous activities no adaptation to the normal Scout training is needed.

Useful training and teaching techniques:

None special.

Additional games and activities equipment:

None.

Deformed or Absent Limbs

The cause of the disability may be disease or accident. The extent of the handicap will vary from a young person having lost a hand or foot to having no natural arms or legs. He may be fitted with artificial limbs operated by mechanical or electronic devices. The only criterion should be that he should participate as fully as possible in all aspects of the life of the Group and, as with any other boy, the Leader's commonsense together with the advice of the parents and the boy's doctor, should prevail.

Speech Defects

Complete lack of speech, usually the result of congenital deafness, is now rare. More common in those who are deaf is the monotonal speech which allows them to communicate with people who know them well but which is difficult for the casual acquaintance to understand. Speech may also be impaired by stammering and difficulties in articulation caused by muscular spasm (e.g. as experienced by spastics).

Although the form and cause may vary, the result will be difficulty in communication and in asking questions. Speech difficulties, especially stammering, tend to increase if extra attention is focused on the boy or if he becomes tired or upset.

The instructor needs to watch the boy's performance with care, to see that he has grasped all processes and is confident about what he is doing. If the boy tries to speak he should be given time to express himself without interruption or anticipation of what he is trying to say; the latter practice can be most irritating to the boy, particularly as the listener often jumps to the wrong conclusion.

The young person may find speaking easier when he is in a group of other boys, when attention will not be focused on him alone.

A pad and pencil can help in a real emergency but should not be too readily available as it may encourage laziness in trying to speak.

Kidney Failure

What it is:

The inability to pass urine.

How it affects young people:

Lack of energy. The eyesight is possibly affected and there may be a difficulty in focusing. There will be a slight yellow discolouration of the complexion. He will be able to do only a very limited amount of exercise.

Boys in chronic renal failure will have to attend hospital for haemodialysis twice or three times per week, which would curtail their Scouting activities.

Education:

Usually at an ordinary school.

Safety and Welfare

Advisable additional facilities:

None.

Points to watch during meetings, activities, etc.:

(a) Bleeding, which can be clearly seen as a bandage is worn on either the arm or the leg.

Any danger of collision with this site must be avoided (e.g. soccer, 'contact' games, etc.)

(b) Excess swelling of the face or ankles, and any complaints of shortness of breath.

Routine First Aid treatment required:

Pressure bandages only, at any time when the *shunt has become damaged and the patient is bleeding.

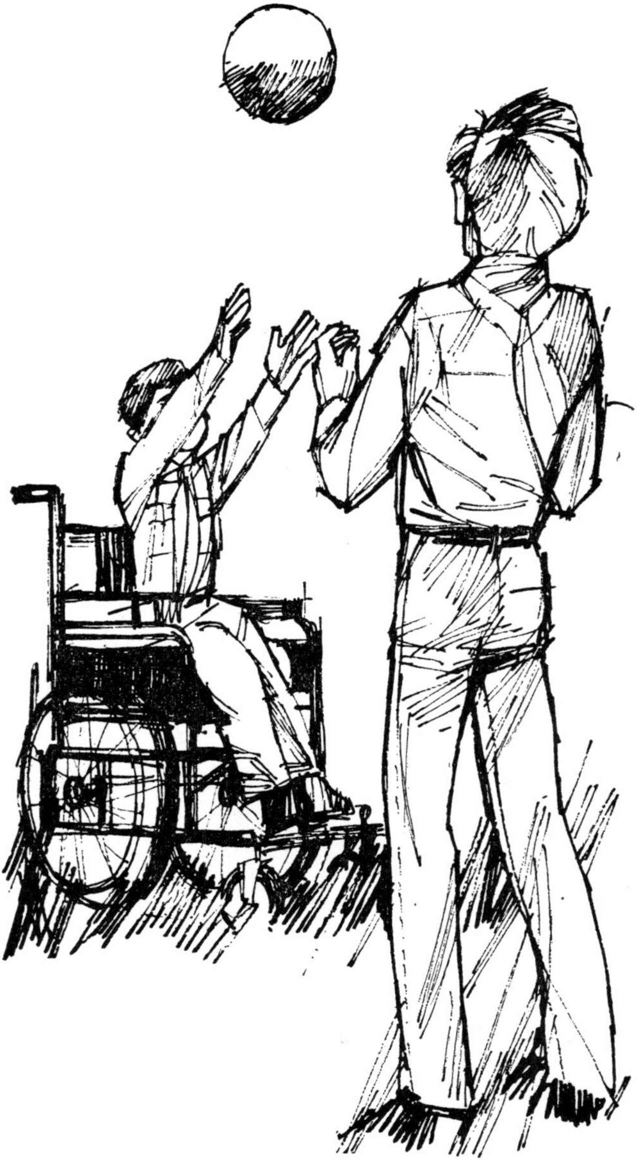

Additional items for the First Aid Kit:
Pressure bandages. Medication supplied by doctor.

Knowledge of Aids and Equipment:
None.

Programme

Activities in which the boy can most likely participate:
Mapping, knotting, signalling, handicraft, nature study, etc.

Activities in which the boy can least likely participate:
Those where physical exertion is required, e.g. strenuous games, climbing, etc.

Useful training and teaching techniques:
Anything which stimulates the brain and interests the boy and which will enable him to feel a useful member of the community and help him to forget his disability.

Additional games and activities equipment:
None in particular.

Reference Material

While there are no relevant publications available as yet, the Renal Unit at Dulwich Hospital (address page 92) or the local Unit will help.

* A vessel tip of teflon is inserted into the arterial and venous arteries to be connected up to the kidney machine during dialysis. The means of connecting these two together to allow normal circulation is done by another silastic tube connected to them and commonly known as a shunt. These are usually bandaged to the patient and taped, but sometimes during activities they are caught by people's shoes or a piece of furniture and bleed. Hence the suggested treatment as before.

CHAPTER 5

"Invisible" Handicaps

Introduction

Everyone knows what it means to be physically ill or crippled but many people do not realise that there are corresponding mental disorders. People who are mentally disordered include those who are mentally ill and those who are mentally subnormal. It is important to understand the difference between the two.

Anyone of any level of intelligence can become mentally ill at any time of life. Most of us occasionally experience minor symptoms of mental disturbance. For example, we feel depressed or afraid for no good reason or are convinced that everyone is against us. We have nightmares during which frightening fantasies become more real to us than reality. Some people are overpowered by such feelings and fantasies, which prevent them from going to work, doing the housekeeping or looking after their children. Such people are considered mentally ill. The chances of recovery from mental illness are good.

The mentally subnormal, on the other hand, are almost always born crippled mentally by the disability of having very limited intelligence. This means that they have great difficulty in learning to walk and talk and can seldom master ordinary school subjects, such as reading, writing and arithmetic. A common type of mental subnormality is 'mongolism'.

There is still a great tendency to confuse intellectual handicap with mental illness. The clear distinction between these two conditions is that intellectual handicaps are not curable and are only amenable to improvement through educational treatment while mental illness is often overcome by suitable treatment, either within society itself or with the aid of doctors, psychiatrists, etc. Those children who suffer from low intelligence and those children who suffer from various kinds of mental illness do not require the same kind of approach in the Scouting situation. For example, many disturbed and maladjusted children have a very high intelligence, which is sometimes one of the reasons why they are disturbed.

Autism

What it is:

There exists a condition – which is probably psychotic based – which is described as autism. Complete agreement on its causes and effects do not exist and clearly much research remains to be undertaken. In general, however, persons suffering this type of handicap find difficulty in relating and interpreting what is seen and what is heard to any sort of rational basis. Their eyes and ears are physically normal.

How it affects young people:

There is a very wide range of handicap in autistic children, depending on the degree of severity of the handicap and the intelligence of the child. Autism leads to isolation in the child because he is unable to communicate. His behaviour may also be inappropriate because he will have difficulty, without special help, of understanding what is happening.

Education:

Autistic children will be found at special boarding schools, special day schools and ordinary schools, depending upon their intelligence and local facilities.

Safety and Welfare

Advisable additional facilities:

For a mildly handicapped child no special precautions need be taken and no special facilities are necessary. For a severely handicapped boy one would have to make sure that he would not be able to wander away. It is not advisable to accept a severely autistic child in an ordinary Group unless someone is prepared to give him their undivided attention.

Points to watch during meetings, activities, etc.:

(a) A severely handicapped autistic child has no sense of *real* danger although he may be frightened of something quite ordinary or a harmless object. He may run across a busy road or climb out of an upstairs window. It is unlikely that the parents of a severely handicapped child would ask him to join the Movement.

Routine First Aid treatment required:

A few autistic children are also epileptic.

Additional items for the First Aid Kit:

None.

Knowledge of Aids or Equipment:

None.

Programme

Activities in which the boy is most likely to be able to participate:

Climbing and practical activities. Although not all autistic children like climbing, many do.

Spheres of activitity in which the boy is least likely to be able to participate:

Those requiring group communication. He will need someone to 'translate' for him.

Useful training and teaching techniques:

It would be helpful if Leaders understood the special language handicap of autistic children. They progress well with individual attention.

Additional games and activities equipment:

Practical equipment requiring no imagination. Simple games, the rules of which are easy to explain to a child who has difficulty in understanding what is said.

Reference Material

The Siege, by Clara Clairborn Park, published Colin Smythe is an excellent book for those knowing nothing of the subject. A publications list is available from the National Society for Autistic Children (address page 93).

Intellectual Handicaps

The handicaps described and explained in the previous chapter are, broadly speaking, 'obvious'. To a large extent the integration of boys with physical handicaps into ordinary Groups is principally a matter of practical consideration. In most instances the handicap can be easily identified or explained, and both Leaders and boys can understand why a boy with physical handicap may not be able to do particular activities or parts of the Section's training programme. There are a great many children who go through life with an invisible handicap. Physically they may be 'sound in wind and limb' but their intellectual or mental capabilities are below average. Just as there is a great difference between a boy who is without one finger and a boy who has lost both his legs, so there are different graduations of intellectual and social handicaps.

Since the implementation of the Education (Handicapped Children) Act 1970 *all* children in England and Wales, including those who are severely sub-normal (with I.Q.'s of below 50-55) come under the Department of Education and Science insofar as their training and education is concerned. No longer can children be referred to as *ineducable,* since the word 'education' covers the development of social competence in all its aspects and does not refer simply to reading, writing and arithmetic.

Although there are three broad categories of intellectual handicap – retarded; educationally sub-normal or slow learner; and the severely sub-normal – the variations in the extent of the handicap within each category are enormous and generalisations are dangerous. In all cases of intellectual handicaps, however, the individual child or young person is often doubly at a disadvantage compared with his contemporaries due to (1) the intellectual handicap itself, and (2) the lack of opportunity to mix with his contemporaries which can heighten his *own* feelings of being 'different' or 'inferior'.

What is intelligence?

Intelligence is an inborn, all round mental power. Slight alterations can be made by environmental influences, although in the main it is determined by experiences. Because intelligence is concerned with the higher mental processes, a child with learning difficulties rarely succeeds with those things which involve the abstract or the theoretical.

The technique of intelligence testing is far from perfect, but the tests do provide the most accurate means known of judging general intelligence, and classifying it as an Intelligence Quotient (I.Q.) for an individual. It is recognised (1) that too much emphasis cannot be placed on the result of one intelligence test and (2) that it would be wrong to read *too* much into an individual's I.Q. However, it can be both helpful and useful because it gives a *guide* to his mental age. For example, you would not expect a Scout of average intelligence, aged 11, to be able to have the understanding of a Scout of average intelligence aged 16. It would, therefore, be quite wrong to expect a boy of 16 who has a *mental age* of 12 to do all that a boy of 16 of average intelligence (whose *mental age* will also be 16) can do. The Scout Association does not lay down a dividing line at a particular level of I.Q. stating that all those 'above' the line can join regular Groups and all those 'below' the line should do their Scouting in Extension Groups. This decision is one for the individual Group to make once they have weighed up all the factors, and have then answered the key question: 'What is in the best interests of the boy?'

What *is* clearly laid down is that the chronological age ranges of the Training Sections must be strictly observed. For example, a boy of 12 who has a mental age of 9 should be a Scout and *not* a Cub Scout.

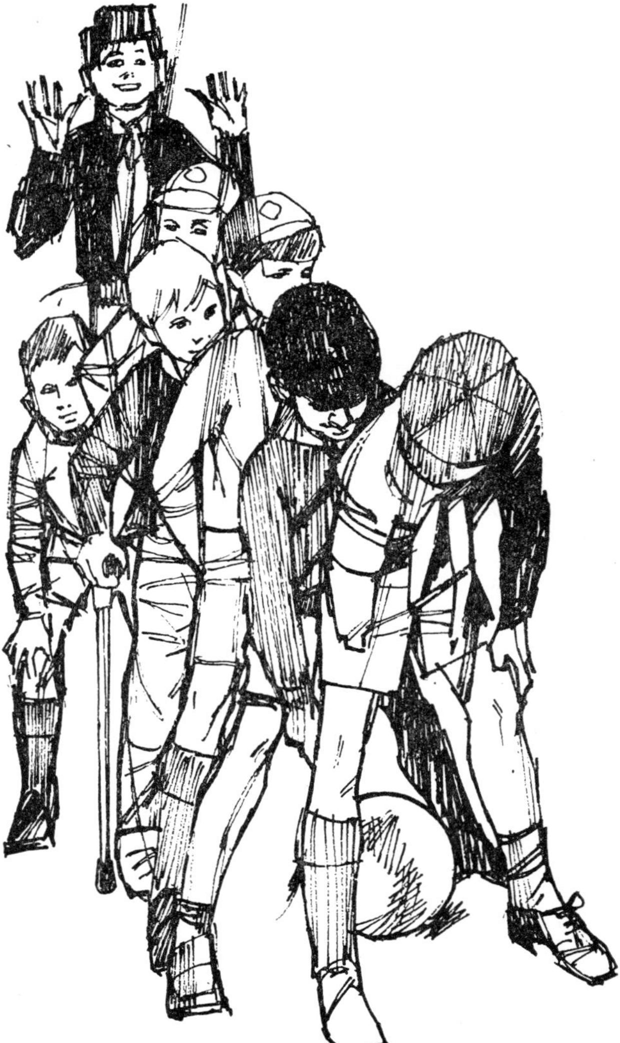

Slow Learners

(also called Educationally Sub-Normal or a child with learning difficulties – we shall refer to them as Slow Learners). The slow learner will always be below average intelligence, but he can learn to live with his handicap and to make his way in society as a stable person.

The characteristics of the Slow Learner

The list below is not 'black and white'. Each slow learner will not have all these characteristics and the extent to which a characteristic is present in an individual will depend on the severity of his handicap.

1. His main difficulties stem from his inability to reason, and to think quickly and logically. All learning processes are difficult. When faced with a problem, the solution of which requires concentration and/or mental agility, he will tend to give up and will not bother to try.
2. He finds listening and concentration hard and tends to expect other people to listen for him, particularly if he cannot keep up with or understand what someone is talking about. He might hear the first word or two of a sentence, 'lose' the next section and pick up again with the last word. He would jump to conclusions of what had been said and either act foolishly or make no attempt to carry out the instructions.
3. His vocabulary is limited, and the more syllables a word has, the less likely he is to understand it. He is unlikely to ask for an explanation of what he does not understand because to do so would be an admission *by himself* of his handicap.
4. 'Abstract' words like left and right, the points of the compass, etc., often will not be understood.
5. Reading is a particularly difficult exercise. He will ignore words which are printed or written in small sized type, lines with lots of words, and pages which have solid text.
6. His manipulative skills in such activities as knotting, lashings, making things, etc, are very restricted and his co-ordination can be poor.
7. He needs constant repetition to remember anything and simple, detailed explanations to ensure some measure of understanding.
8. He can become easily frustrated and seeks attention either by exhibitionism or being physically aggressive. He is living in a world in which everyone he meets does things better than he can, while he is mentally blind to much that is going on around him. For example, a journey into town does not give him as much stimulation as other children because the

slow learner sees advertisements, posters, signposts, etc., only as patterns and he makes little or no attempt to decipher their meaning.

Because he cannot meet the demands of society he becomes baffled, frustrated, upset and disorientated.

Where the Slow Learner is Educated

It is most important to restate that there are different degrees of learning handicaps just as there are different degrees of illness or physical handicap. Some children can continue in a remedial class at an ordinary school, some are educated in a Day Special School, some in a Boarding Special School, and some require hospital treatment.

Special Notes

1. It is estimated that 10% of the school population are slow learners and that by 1972 at least one million children were in this category.

2. If a child attends a Special School it will be known that he is a slow learner. However, where the slow learner is educated in a remedial class of an ordinary school, the fact that he *is* a slow learner will not necessarily be known to an 'outsider'. Neither the child nor his parents are likely to be readily forthcoming with this *vital* fact.

Scouting and the Slow Learner

Scouting can be advantageous to the slow learner because it:

(a) enables him to make the best use of his practical abilities and physical skills,

(b) helps him to see himself as an equal part of an accepted section of society; his uniform not only positively identifies him with it, but also gives him the chance to minimise his handicap,

(c) stimulates a desire to do and learn, and encourage him to try things which previously he had automatically rejected as impossible.

Scouting can be disadvantageous to the slow learner because it:

(a) places considerable emphasis on progress and achievement, and the lack of progress, compared with his friends, could make him even more aware of his handicap,

(b) does have competitive elements with, for example, inter-Six and inter-Patrol competitions: his slowness or repeated making of mistakes could cause resentment in even the most well-intentioned and understanding Cub Scout in his Six or Scout in his Patrol.

The Slow Learner in the ordinary Group

Chapter 1 (No One is Perfect) describes the variety of individuals who can be found in any Group. The boys in an ordinary Group will often have I.Q.'s ranging from below 75 (an I.Q. of 75 means that the intellectual age of the individual is 75% of his physical age) to over 120. Because the slow learner has an invisible handicap the Scouters may not realise that they do have slow learners in their Section . . . until it is too late. If the Leaders do not recognise the reasons for a boy's lack of ability, and if the boy does not make personal progress because of an unawareness on the Leader's part, the boy may leave, usually without giving the *real* reason. He will not say that he cannot cope with the pace of the Section.

Identifying the Slow Learner

1. The reason for the Scouter knowing that a boy *is* a slow learner is so that he can better *understand* the boy as an individual, and make any necessary provision for him to enjoy his Scouting. It is *not* to set him apart from the other boys, nor to 'categorise' him as a member of the Extension Branch.
2. Scouting has always been a partnership between the boy, the other boys, the Scouters and the parents. *Sometimes,* but probably not often enough, the boy's teachers are also brought into the partnership.
3. The Cub Scouter who thinks that he or she has a slow learner in their Pack would be wise to make an informal contact with the boy's school to ascertain his level of intelligence. Early 'diagnosis' will be of benefit to all concerned as this knowledge will not only enable the Scouters to help the Cub Scout make progress within the limits of his capabilities but could also be a – and perhaps *the* – critical factor in ensuring the boy's continuing enjoyment of Scouting in the Troop and ultimately in the Venture Scout Unit.

Integrating the Slow Learner in the ordinary Group

*'Recent developments in unstreamed schools seem to show that backward children benefit from remaining in their peer group, particularly if they receive special additional help in basic subjects.'**

This principle is equally applicable to Scouting. Those boys who attend ordinary schools can be (and already are) successfully integrated into ordinary Groups. As long as a Scouter *knows* that a boy *is* a slow learner he will have an idea of what the boy's capabilities are. With patience and understanding a slow learner whose handicap is not too severe can be given, and receive, the best of Scouting.

**Pseudo-Backwardness* by A. E. Tansley, a chapter in *Time Unredeemable* published by the Schoolmaster Publishing Co. Ltd.

Aids to Training Slow Learners

(Many of these suggestions are already used by Scouters, whether or not they realise they have slow learners in their Section.)

(a) Give additional, individual instruction where a boy is finding difficulty.

(b) Use games and visual aids as much as possible.

(c) The slow learner needs more attention and repetition than others, and once having learnt a skill or activity he needs constant revision.

(d) He will find great difficulty in expressing himself in writing, but can be encouraged to develop his powers of observation by answering questions one at a time.

(e) Written instructions must be in a script which they can read and in a language which they can understand.

(f) Avoid giving a boy with a speech defect activities involving verbal messages.

(g) After verbal and/or written instructions it may be necessary to get someone (a Scouter, Instructor, Patrol Leader, etc.) to do the project as an insurance of comprehension.

The Severely Sub-normal

Those children who are severely sub-normal are unable to qualify for membership of the Scout Movement because their intellectual age is so young that they cannot have even the simplest understanding of the Promise and the Law.

This does not mean that Scouting ignores these youngsters. There is much scope, particularly for older Scouts and Venture Scouts, to plan and run games and activities through a club which is sponsored by a school, hospital or organisation but which is not a 'formal' part of The Scout Association.

There are a growing number of voluntary organisations providing special provision for the severely sub-normal, which supplement the statutory social services, among which are:

The National Association for Mental Health (address page 92) which has nearly seventy local associations in England and Wales. It sponsors and organises many activities to help the mentally ill and the mentally handicapped.

The National Elfrida Rathbone Society (address page 92) through local committees assists the educationally handicapped in many ways including youth clubs for junior and senior school children and young people starting employment to give them social experience and self confidence in new situations and support them as they move from school to job; involving the community in the welfare of the educationally handicapped; encouraging other local organisations to

befriend them; spreading information and arousing interest.
The National Society for Mentally Handicapped Children (address page 92) whose objects are to increase the public awareness of the problems of the mentally handicapped so as to secure provision for them commensurate with their needs.
The National Federation of Gateway Clubs (address page 93).

Social Handicaps

Socially Deprived Children

It is vital to appreciate that a *retarded* child does not have an intellectual handicap in the sense that it has been defined in the previous section. He is medically normal but *appears* to be of below average intelligence. In fact he has all the 'equipment' but, for such reasons as lack of schooling, lack of stimulation, poor environment with a background of moral, social or educational starvation, he has been denied the opportunities of normal development. Under favourable environmental changes, a retarded child is able to catch up and reach the norms. Because of this, Scouting can play a beneficial part in what amounts to the child's rehabilitation. Whether or not these children are educated in a special school, they also need outside school in order to make social relationships and to have the enjoyable and enriching leisure time that most people take for granted. Social experience will give them confidence to cope with the responsibilities and tensions of adult life.

Maladjustment

Maladjusted children are emotionally inadequate. They grow up in a society to which they want to belong but to which they cannot adjust. The root cause of many cases of maladjustment is the lack of a stable family environment. Scouting may possibly help to provide a stable society in which the boy is accepted but it is impossible to lay down any general guide lines.
Boys who are severely socially ill-adapted or with character troubles very rarely wish to become members of a Scout Group.
The problems of children who are mildly maladjusted are psychological ones and do not require adaptation of Scout programmes or training (including games) for this would be psychologically dangerous. There should be a place for these boys as individuals like the rest of the Group and not

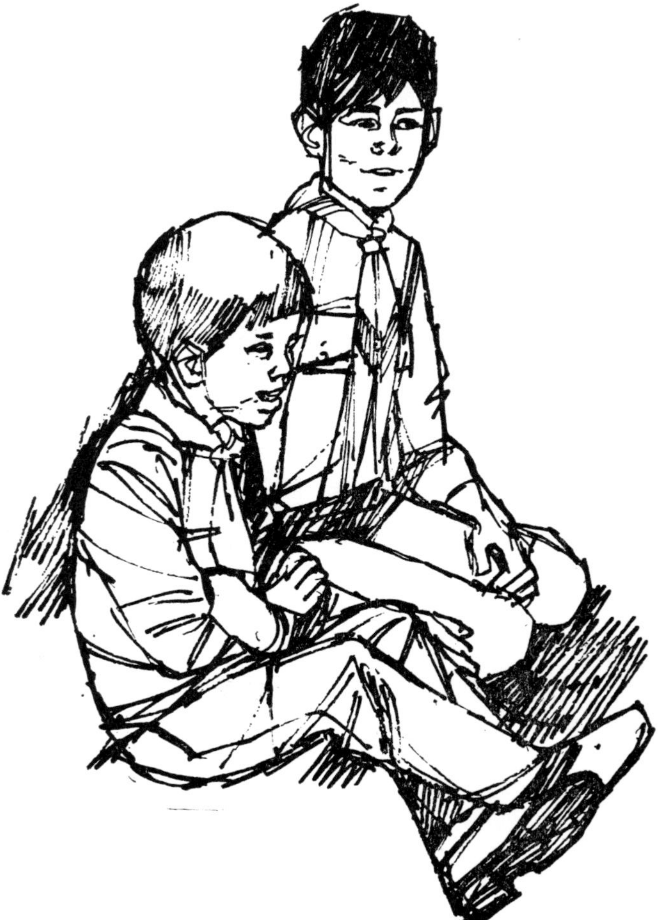

as categories in an ordinary Scout Group and there should be no segregation.

Characteristics of the maladjusted boy

1. He is not really socially acceptable to his contemporaries which can lead to tensions on both sides.
2. He has a poor sense of honour and will let people down on many occasions.

The maladjusted boy in the ordinary Group

The right Leader with the right Group can do much to help the individual maladjusted boy, but the problems of coping with the boy are immense. A Scouter who is considering taking a maladjusted boy should preferably first see the District Extension Adviser, and then have discussions with the boy's parents and/or the professional staff of the Child Guidance Clinic which the boy attends.

Cub Scout Pack: it is not recommended that maladjusted boys should be members of ordinary Cub Packs.

Scout Troop: after the initial enquiries the Patrol Leaders' Council should freely discuss the problem and due weight be given to their opinions and conclusions.

Venture Scout Unit: the decision rests with the Executive Committee.

Extension Groups in Special Schools

(see also Chapter 7).

A large proportion of maladjusted boys are educated at residential schools. The basic principles of Scouting and the Patrol system can sometimes enable a boy to adjust to a small part of society and from this may come acceptance of general social principles. Integration of a boy into an ordinary Group when he leaves school may help to bridge the gap between the anti-social boy and society.

CHAPTER 6

Recruitment

Introduction

It is worth noting that not all boys – whether or not they have a handicap – will want to become *Scouts.* Also, while The Scout Association is one of the youth organisations which does provide for a boy with a handicap, there are others! This chapter is primarily concerned with what can be done, and how it should be done.

There are five principal ways in which a boy with a handicap is – or can be – introduced to Scouting.

1. Often boys who are already Cub Scouts, Scouts or Venture Scouts know where boys with a handicap live – next door, down the road or in a nearby street. Your boys may approach you or, by 'planting the seed' of the idea of having a boy with a handicap in your Section, your boys might well find one.
2. By the parents of a boy with a handicap asking you if you can take their son into your Section.
3. By an officer of a statutory or voluntary organisation (for example, the Social Services Officer, the Probation Officer, the Secretary of the local Branch of a Voluntary Society) making an enquiry.
4. By a regular Group wanting to extend Scouting to boys with a handicap without having any particular boy or boys in mind.
5. The District or County Extension Adviser may wish to find a place for a boy.
6. By starting a Pack and/or a Troop in a Special School.

This book is primarily concerned with 1-5, which is the concern of all Scouters, and these points are considered in more detail in this chapter. It is, however, imperative that it should be clearly understood that starting a Group in a Special School involves a different procedure to starting an ordinary Group: this procedure is clearly laid down by The Scout Association in *Policy, Organisation and Rules.* Briefly, the normal pattern for the formation of an ordinary Group is for the District Commissioner and the District Scout Council to decide that a Group *will* be formed and to send the regi-

stration forms to Headquarters. When consideration is being given to the formation of a Group in a Special School, permission must first be sought and obtained from Headquarters. When boys leave school they have the opportunity of Further Education and they should be encouraged to join the Venture Scouts.
Chapter 7 describes the Extension Group.

Paving the Way

The following paragraphs contain some suggestions for paving the way for Scouting with the handicapped in a regular Group. They are practical ideas which could be included in *any* Group's programme at any time whether or not a boy with a handicap has applied to join. They are not a chronological sequence of events and activities, all of which have to be completed before a boy with a handicap can be accepted. You can take them, leave them, put them in a different order or make a selection as you wish. Some, particularly those marked with an asterisk, will enable those Groups which cannot, at a particular point in time, accept boys with handicaps to gain an insight into Scouting with the handicapped and an awareness of what can be done and what is being done.

**CONTACT YOUR DISTRICT OR COUNTY EXTENSION ADVISER.* He will know what *is* being done, and what *could* be done in your area. He could be asked to:

(a) Take part in a 'round table' discussion with *all* Scouters in the Group.

(b) Give a talk (preferably illustrated with slides or films) on Scouting with the handicapped to any or all of the following:– Pack Meeting, Troop Meeting, Unit Meeting, Group Council. The Group or District Annual General Meeting also provides an ideal platform (particularly if the boys are present) as it gives an excellent opportunity for the dissemination of information and a full discussion with *all* those who could be involved – boys, Scouters, lay officers, parents and others interested in the life of the Group.

(c) Put you in touch with a Group in a Special School or a Group which already has boys with handicaps (see Joint Meetings page 61).

**ASKING THE BOYS.* No matter how enthusiastic the Leaders may be, the success or failure of integrating a boy with a handicap will depend to a great extent on the attitude of the *Scouts* already in the Group. Young people can tend to reject an idea or a proposition on principle when they are presented by adults with a *fait accompli.* Yet, when actively involved in planning and decision-making, they are not only capable of deep thought and understanding but also are often rational and practical. Obviously Cub Scouts require far more 'guidance by adult leadership' than Scouts: Venture Scouts become or are adults and the Unit Executive is responsible for its own affairs.

Cub Scouts.

Boys can be very cruel to other boys, though in most cases they do not intend to be. It is quite natural for them to act first and think afterwards. For example, they will mimic deformities and, in the heat of inter-Six competitions, can come out with scathing comments (and sometimes use physical means of settling disputes) which may *temporarily* hurt another boy. These situations are ones which the Leaders can sort out quickly. For a boy with a handicap these outbursts could do irreparable damage to his relationships with the other boys. In spite of – or perhaps because of – this, Cubs do have large reservoirs of common humanity which is tapped by the Leaders giving them their trust and having confidence in them.

THE SIXERS' COUNCIL is not a decision-making body and the Leader must retain the right to 'veto' suggestions. The Council is not, however, a platform from which the Leader merely issues 'orders'. Its effectiveness is bound to vary between one Pack and another. One thing is certain. Those Packs which do have a *working* Sixers' Council and thus actively involve the older boys in the running of the Pack are more likely to be able to accept a boy with a handicap.

THE PACK. What do the Cubs *imagine* having a boy with a handicap in the Pack would be like? A full Pack Meeting with the Scouters leading the discussion will not be particularly useful because:

1. The Cubs, quite naturally, are likely to say what they think the Leader would *like* them to say, rather than what they really feel.

2. The shy and more reserved boys will say little or nothing.

One way to overcome these factors would be to tell the Sixers that you want them to find out what their Six think about having a boy with a handicap in the Pack. To help them 'chair' their Six Meetings give each Sixer a message along these lines:

> Akela has asked us to imagine that a boy who is crippled and can therefore only get about in a wheelchair has asked if he can become a Cub Scout in our Pack. Akela would like to know exactly what we, as a Six, think of the idea and, if we were asked to have

a handicapped boy in our Six, whether we would accept him and how we could help him make the most of being a Cub.

SOME QUESTIONS YOU MIGHT ASK IF DISCUSSION DRIES UP:– How would having a boy with a handicap in the Pack affect the Pack programme? What extra things do you think we would have to do to help him? Do you think that boys with handicaps would enjoy Cub Scouting in an ordinary Pack?

Make it quite clear to the Sixers that the Cubs should be encouraged to say exactly what they think. Let each Six have a meeting lasting only 3-5 minutes *without* a Scouter being present, and then each Six should give a brief report to the Pack on what was said. An ideal way of doing this project is with a tape recorder, thus freeing the Sixer from the difficult job of making notes and remembering what was said. What the boys say will provide a sound basis for a short general discussion on Scouting with the handicapped and the opportunity to correct any misconceptions they might have expressed. This sort of approach will give the boys a much greater sense of involvement because it encourages them to think in real and personal terms, rather than in theoretical or abstract ideas.

Scouts.

Compared with Cub Scouting there are a number of important differences in the approach to Scouting with the handicapped in the Troop under this heading of *Asking the Boys.*

1. The Patrol System. Its constitution and application is fully described in *The Patrol Leader's Handbook, The Scout Handbook,* and *The Scout Leader's Handbook.* In the context of this book, suffice it to say that the Scouts must (not should) not only be asked for their opinions but also must be allowed to make their own decisions.

2. The Patrol Leaders and older Scouts will have a much greater part to play in the Scouting life of the boy with the handicap.

3. Unlike the Cub Scout Pack which has only one source of recruitment (direct), the Troop has two (from the Cub Scout Pack and direct). It is therefore vital that the Troop as a whole and the Patrol Leaders' Council in particular is kept fully informed, and is encouraged to voice its opinions on any proposals under consideration for the Pack which will, sooner or later, affect the Troop.

Venture Scouts.

Nothing need be added to what has been said, as Venture Scouts are mature enough to read this book as though they were Leaders. (Many are already.) *Venture Scouting* and *Notes for Venture Scout Leaders* include sections on Scouting with the handicapped *within* the Unit, within the Pack and Troop, and within the community. Mixed Ranger Guide/ Venture Scout Units afford even greater opportunities for working with the handicapped.

**SEE FOR YOURSELVES.* This does *not* mean a commission of enquiry to go and have a look at *Scouts* with handicaps as though they were odd or different. Lack of pomp and formality are essential if you are to see the boys as they really are. You know what a different bunch of characters the Cubs or Scouts in your Section can be when they are forewarned of a visit by an important person – often they either shut up like clams and become overawed with shyness, or they behave as though butter wouldn't melt in their mouths.

An ideal way of introducing Cub Scouts and Scouts (as well as Scouters) to Scouting with the handicapped is by a joint meeting either with an Extension Group or with an ordinary Group which has already successfully integrated boys with handicaps. A joint meeting gives ideal opportunities for boys and Leaders to meet, talk, mix and *participate* in a programme and atmosphere well known to all concerned.

In any event these joint meetings, particularly between ordinary Groups and Extension Groups, are mutually valuable in themselves whether or not the ordinary Group can accept boys with handicaps. It gives the boys from the ordinary Group a wider appreciation of what Scouting is all about, and will give a real and positive meaning to the brotherhood of Scouting to the boys with handicaps.

**LEADER 'SWOPPING'.* It is said that 'a change is as good as a rest'. The occasional 'swopping' of some (but not all) of the Leaders between an ordinary Group and an Extension Group to assist in the planning and execution of a Section Meeting can act as a stimulus and be mutually advantageous to both Groups.

**OCCASIONAL ADDITIONAL ASSISTANCE.* Scouters, Venture Scouts and older Scouts (particularly the latter two) can be of great help to Extension Groups on expeditions, outings and camps where additional assistance is always required. The boys and young men in the training Sections could be encouraged to look to their brother Scouts with handicaps for the 'Service' sections of the training schemes. After all, charity begins at home.

Dual Membership

Just as many boys who go away to school or university

maintain links with Groups in their home-town during the holidays, so boys with handicaps who attend special boarding schools could be encouraged to join a local Group during the holidays. However, it must be pointed out that while boys in boarding schools were Cub Scouts at home *before* they went away, most of the boys with handicaps first became *Scouts* at their Special School. Furthermore, a large number of boys with handicaps start at their special boarding school before the age of eight.

Dual membership has obvious benefits for the boy with the handicap. For the ordinary Group which cannot cope with a boy with a handicap all year round, it could enable it to make a real and worthwhile contribution, without overstretching its manpower or resources. Because the Special School is often some distance from the boy's home, liaison with the District or County Extension Adviser will probably be needed to find out where these boys live but do not forget to ask your own boys, as they may know of a boy with a handicap living in their street.

Getting Yourself Prepared

In most cases a Scouter is already prepared (in this sense) to accept boys with a handicap. As has been said earlier – but it is worth repeating – many (if not most) Groups already have boys who could be 'classified' as handicapped.

Six areas of further preparation which could be considered are:

1. Training

The Scout Association: Training courses on Extension Activities are run at Gilwell Park and other centres. The courses are designed to meet the specialised needs of Scouters (of all Sections) working with the handicapped and to introduce other Leaders to the problems affecting the integration of boys with handicaps into regular Troops and Packs. Details of these courses are published in *Scouting* and are available from the Programme and Training Department of Scout Headquarters.

Other organisations also run courses and conferences.

2. First Aid

From Chapters 4 and 5 it will be noted that in all but a few instances only routine first aid will be needed. In the remainder the boy's parents and/or doctor will be the person most suitable to contact. No approach should be made to the doctor without the prior written consent of the boy's parent or guardian, and the physician will not, of course, divulge

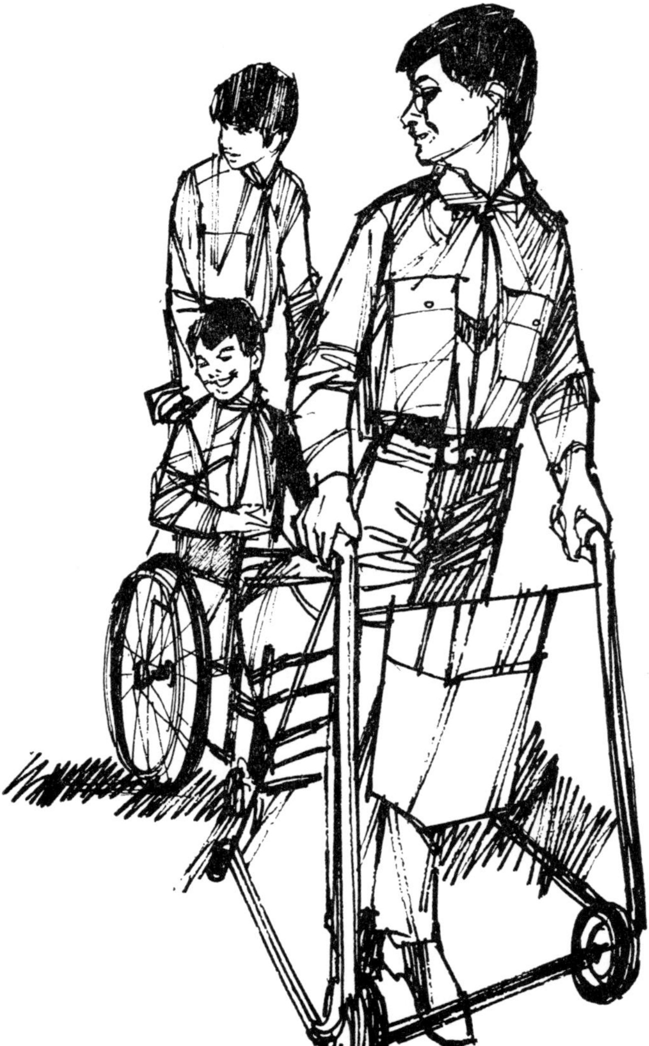

confidential information. Equally, any information given must be regarded as confidential.

3. Additional Assistance

Additional adult help for the Section may or may not be required depending on the nature and severity of the handicap. Among those who might be approached are – the District and/or County Extension Adviser; the Group Supporters' Association; the Society or Societies dealing with the handicap (many have local branches); the Social Services Department of the Local Authority; the local Youth Services office; parents; Rotary; Round Table, etc.

4. Additional Facilities

From Chapters 4 and 5 it will have been seen that additional facilities will not usually be needed. However, if adaptations are required contact the Social Services Department and/or the Education Department of the Local Authority for advice. They may also assist in the financing of any necessary alterations.

5. The Boy's Mechanical and/or Other Aids

(e.g. wheelchair, artificial limbs, crutches, etc.)
Where necessary a knowledge of such things as wheelchair management is necessary for the safety and welfare of the young person.

Ask the boy himself.

Most boys with handicaps who use mechanical aids will be able to tell you what to do and how to do it . . . and will be delighted to do so. One of the leading medical research scientists working on physical aids for the disabled states: 'The range of mechanical aids is extremely wide and the amount of space which would be required to give even background information on, for example, powered artificial limbs would be out of all proportion to the number of children who might become *Scouts.* Both adult leaders and boys should be aware of the need to understand their colleagues' equipment as well as their handicap . . . The leaders – and perhaps the boys – should contact the unit which has issued the equipment and . . . the parents of those with handicaps would be only to pleased to help in this . . . No supplying clinic would present any difficulties in arranging for instruction . . . This would be far better than any treatment of isolated examples of aids, particularly as the design of these and the general approach to them does vary from area to area and no treatment could be comprehensive.'

6. The Scout Training Programmes

There are no such things as 'alternative badge requirements' for boys with handicaps. The *Scout* Badge is the basic requirement for membership of the Scout Movement and anything less is unacceptable. Wherever possible the *Scout* with a handicap should meet the requirements of a particular badge.

Where it is not possible for a boy to attain the standard or complete a project in a reasonable time, or where it is likely to aggravate a particular handicap, it is the Leader of the Section who decides the need for, and the requirements of, any amending badge conditions. The Leader can always ask the District Extension Adviser to help.

When devising equivalent requirements for a badge, equal challenge and the need for comparable effort should be considered as for the existing ones. They should also meet the same purpose with the same expectancy of success.

Some *suggestions* as to possible amended badge requirements are given in Appendix I but it cannot be over emphasised that the responsibility for amending badge requirements rests fairly and squarely on the Section Leader using his own judgement and his personal knowledge of the boy . . . it is not the requirement itself that matters but rather the effort the boy puts into it and the satisfaction he derives from achieving something.

What You Will Need To Know About The Boy

The Physical Education Adviser of a large Society for the handicapped writes: 'I feel that the main defects of any scheme in which the handicapped are invited to join are integration and equal participation. As soon as special arrangements start being made (even special type interviews with parents) then the handicapped boy or girl starts feeling "special" and apart . . . the battle is almost lost before it has begun.

'These are just boys who want to join a Scout Group and should be treated as any other boy. When a Leader is confronted with three so-called "normal" boys he does not worry that one can run 100 metres in 12 seconds, another cannot swim or tie knots, or that the third cannot kick a ball. He takes these boys and uses his own experience and intelligence to treat each boy on his merits, and sets each boy tasks and standards within his maximum capacity . . . he stretches the boy as best he can . . .'

Recruitment

When any boy wishes to join the Movement (in whichever Section) it is *normal* practice to ask the parent or guardian to complete an application form along the following lines:

NONSUCH SCOUT GROUP

I would like my son/ward to join the above Group.
FULL NAME .... DATE OF BIRTH ....
ADDRESS ....
TELEPHONE NUMBER (if any) ....
SCHOOL ....
RELIGION ....
BRIEF DETAILS OF ANY DISABILITIES ....
....
Parent or Guardian's Signature .... Date ....

It is *normal* practice for Scouters to visit parents to establish a firm foundation of relationships with them to enlist their support, understanding, interest and involvement in their son's Scouting activities. It is *normal* practice to find out what restrictions there may be on activities for such ailments as hay fever.

There is no difference in procedure when dealing with an application from a boy with a handicap. Using your common-sense as a judge you may require more information in the interests of the boy. For example, if the physical handicap is relatively severe you may need to know (1) what he is not allowed to do (NOT a list of permissible activities), (2) whom to contact in an emergency (e.g. parent, doctor, hospital, etc.), (3) correct medication which needs to be administered.

Where the handicap is of an intellectual nature it is helpful to have some idea of the boy's abilities and difficulties and the circumstances that affect these. It is not always possible to gain detailed information from medical sources but much can be gleaned from the parents, the boy's teachers and from the boy himself. People are often reluctant to question a boy directly, as they do not want to focus attention on his handicap or to cause him embarrassment. However, it is likely that he has already come to terms with his limitations and will be prepared to discuss or indicate what he can and and cannot do. It must, of course, be borne in mind that the boy may have been over-protected or may be reluctant to attempt new tasks for fear of failure, in which case he may underestimate his capacity but may respond surprisingly when presented with a challenge.

Where a boy joins a Scout Group based on his special school, it is reasonable to suppose that the situation is such that his particular difficulties can be catered for in regard to environment, equipment and special instruction.

CHAPTER 7

The Extension Group

To Begin With . . .

1. Whenever possible and practicable boys who want to be *Scouts* should do their Scouting in ordinary Groups, whether they live at home or are educated at special day schools or special boarding schools.
2. In the main, Extension Groups are formed in those hospitals or special schools where it is not possible for the boys to join local Groups by reason of the hospital's or school's geographical location, or where in the general interests of the boys' health, education or welfare, it is not advisable for the boys to do their week-by-week Scouting in a local Group. In the larger urban areas it may be advantageous to establish an open Extension Group, especially where all or most of the special schools are day schools.
3. As this book is primarily concerned with extending Scouting to boys with handicaps in *non*-Extension Groups, this chapter on Extension Groups will be brief.

Starting an Extension Group

When the possibility of starting Scouting in a special school is first considered (whether by a member of the staff, or by a Scouter who is not on the staff) it must not be automatically assumed that a Group can be formed. The A.C.C. (Extension Activities) or County Extension Adviser must be informed. He or she makes some preliminary enquiries, and if these suggest that a Group might be formed within a school, the Programme and Training Department of Headquarters must be consulted immediately, and certainly *before* registration forms are submitted. No Section of a Group will be approved by the Headquarters Commissioner for Extension Activities unless he is satisfied with the result of the enquiries.

Minimum Standards

A Section of an Extension Group, when applying for initial

registration, must comply with the requirements of the Minimum Standards Scheme.

Capitation Fees

Registered Extension Groups pay the usual Capitation Fees, but, in consultation with the District Extension Adviser, a Group may, under special circumstances, apply through the District Commissioner for partial or total exemption by Headquarters.

Leadership

Successful Scouting in the Extension Group in the special school is based on the co-ordination, co-operation and combination of the 'medical' and 'teaching' expertise of the school staff on the one hand, and the Scouting skills of the Scouters on the other. There is no reason why Scouters and Instructors should not be members of the staff (as they are in other school Groups), but there is also no reason why, *with the permission of the Headmaster* (who is usually the sponsoring authority), a person who is not a teacher at the school should not be a Scouter in an Extension Group *providing* (and this is most important) he knows, understands and accepts the teaching methods which are being used in that particular school. For example, sign language is rarely used today for instructing children who are deaf or partially deaf, and an 'outside' Scouter using sign language might well undo the very things that the staff have been teaching.

Programme

Basically, the programme of training and activities is no different from any other Scout Group. Certain areas may need to be amended to suit individual boys but, with ingenuity and imagination, only the minimum alterations are required. As far as the training schemes are concerned, it is the Section Leader who decides what amendments need to be made to particular badge requirements. He bases his decision on his personal knowledge of the individual boy, though he may if *he* wishes, seek the advice of the District Extension Adviser.

Every opportunity should be taken to enable the boys in an Extension Group to meet other Scouts and to participate as fully as possible in District, County, National and International events and activities. Equally, the value of Scouters in Extension Groups seeing Scouting in action in other Groups cannot be over-emphasised.

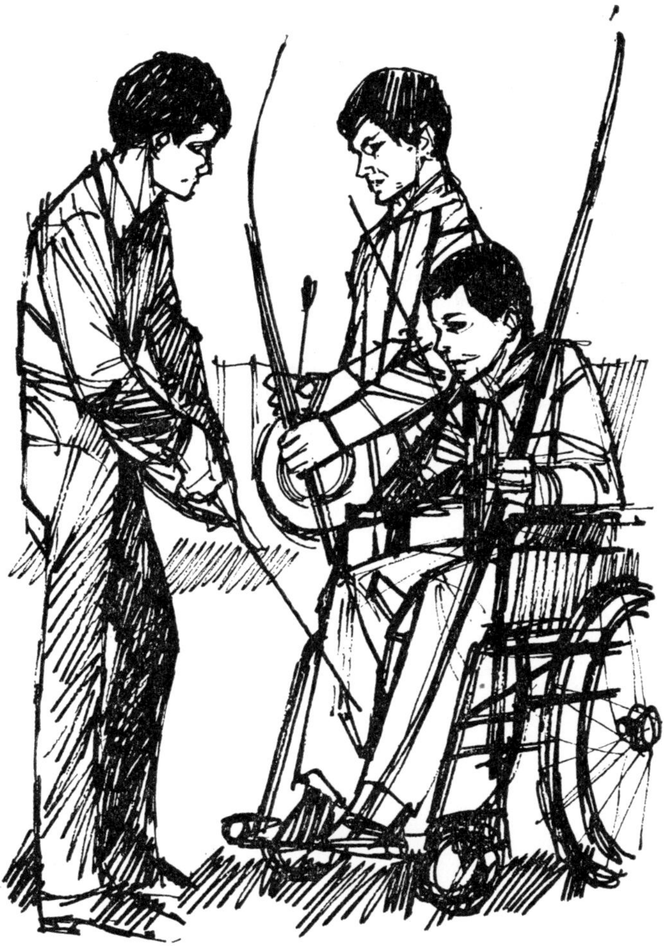

The Educationally Handicapped Boy in a Boarding Special School

Children who receive their education in the boarding special school have undoubtedly generous opportunities for development. Broadly speaking the boarding special school achieves some outstanding successes with their children since the school is specifically designed to meet their needs to the full.

Regularity of routine, meals and occupations stimulate the feeling of security, thus enabling good human relationships and a high standard of personal, physical and spiritual education.

Much that these schools achieve can also be accomplished by Scouting bearing in mind that the principal aims are to assist the children towards personal adequacy and social competency.

The educationally handicapped boy, especially if his handicap is severe enough for him to need boarding placement, is probably happier Scouting in an Open or Sponsored Extension Group dealing specifically with this one handicap.

The meetings can be set to their pace where the techniques used will be accepted by all.

The maintaining of 'live' contact with other Groups would be advisable or the Extension Activities could become a section of an existing Group where automatic Group contact could be offered.

CHAPTER 8

Outdoor Activities and Camping

Much of the appeal of Scouting for a boy is its emphasis on outdoor activities. A boy with a handicap wants to have just as many opportunities to enjoy, explore, learn about and discover the great outdoors as any boy who joins the Movement.

Wherever physically and medically possible and practicable *Scouts* with handicaps should do their Scouting 'on location'. Some suggestions and 'guide lines' for amending badge requirements in the training programme for those with particular physical handicaps are given in Appendix I. The same principle, that it is the boy's Leader who (in consultation with whomever he thinks advisable – parents, medical opinion, etc.) decides whether an amending badge requirement is needed and what it is to be, applies to outdoor activities and camping.

All the usual 'Rules' laid down in *Policy, Organisation and Rules* for such activities as hiking, swimming, camping, etc., apply, as well as any additional rules which may be made by the Section Leader based upon his commonsense, and knowledge of the boy and his handicap.

Physically Handicapped

A. Cub Scouts

(a) Outdoor Activities

Subject only to the limitations of the boy's handicap and any safety precautions, Cubs should participate as much as possible in all Pack outdoor activities. They should not be so surrounded with so many *additional* rules and regulations that it becomes impossible for them to do anything for themselves.

WITHIN THE TRAINING PROGRAMME. All outdoor activities must involve some element of risk. Some examples:

Bronze Arrow 'Feats of Skill' – Climb at least 3 metres (10 feet) up a tree or rope – *any* Cub Scout *could* fall out of the tree or down the rope.

Silver Arrow 'Swimming' – anyone *could* drown in a bowl of water.

Gold Arrow 'Out-of-Doors' – Find the way over a course using a compass – *any* Cub Scout can get lost.
Just because there is some element of risk, it does not mean that the activities are not undertaken. The risks are reduced by training (teaching safety precautions and giving practical demonstrations), practice and experience (doing under supervision), and commonsense on the part of the Leaders and the boys.
Subject to the opening paragraphs of this Chapter, Cub Scouts with physical handicaps should be allowed, and encouraged, to participate as fully as possible in outdoor activities. Let the boy prove to himself (and to the Leaders) what he can do, and not simply tackle those things which his Leaders imagine he can do.

EXPEDITIONS: If a Cub Scout with a handicap cannot complete the entire programme for an expedition either because of the nature of his handicap or the mechanical aids or equipment he uses, do what you can to enable him to participate as fully as possible. A few ideas:
– Plan the route so he can cover a section or two with the Pack (transport will be needed for the 'putting down' and 'pick up' points).
– Give him a number of useful, interesting and practical activities (not something to keep him occupied) on the planning and execution of the expedition. He can do these while the other Cubs are doing the things which he cannot do. For example, he could: help prepare a meal or games for the Pack at a rendezvous point; assist in laying a trail; set a competition regarding the natural or other features of the 'lunch' site for the rest of the Pack to do when they arrive.

(b) Visits

The principal point here is to ensure that the person with whom arrangements for a visit are being made is aware that there are boys with handicaps in the Group. It would be most unfortunate if the Pack had arranged to visit somewhere and upon arrival it was discovered that, for one reason or another, the boy with the handicap had to be excluded.

(c) Pack Holidays and Camping

There is no reason why a Cub Scout with a handicap should not go on a Pack Holiday or camp although, depending on the nature and severity of the handicap, certain additional considerations will need to be made. Some hints and suggestions are given in the section on 'Camping' under Scouts and Venture Scouts and these can be adapted, where necessary, to suit the requirements of the Cub Scout Pack.

B. Scouts and Venture Scouts

(a) Outdoor Activities, Expeditions, etc.

Similar considerations to those mentioned for Cub Scouts apply equally to the older boy and young man, though they will, of course, need to be amended to suit the more advanced requirements of the Scout and Venture Scout Sections. As many more of the requirements for the Scout and Venture Scout Progress Schemes involve outdoor activities, this subject is adequately covered in the Leaders' *Handbooks* and in *Programme Planning in the Scout Troop*. It is worth noting, however, that the older Scout or Venture Scout with a handicap is often ideally suited to help in the planning stages of activities and expeditions even if he is unable to fully participate in the event itself. Scribe or Secretary; time keeper; quartermaster; route planning, etc., – these are just a few of the *necessary* and *vital* ingredients to adventurous activities which the boy with a handicap can do, and, in so doing, it will give him the satisfaction of having helped other members of the Troop or Unit to achieve something, even if the activity itself is physically beyond him. Equally important is the fact that, just because the boy with a handicap cannot undertake a particular outdoor activity (e.g. rock climbing) it must never be assumed that he cannot participate in any outdoor activities. For example, many boys who have difficulty in getting about on land, take to the water like fish and are very proficient swimmers, leading to such activities as canoeing and sailing.

(b) Camping

Like any Scout or Venture Scout, the boy with a handicap will *want* to go to camp, though some may have more than the usual natural apprehension experienced by other boys going away to camp, particularly when it is for the first time. The detailed planning and execution for a camp as far as campcraft and Scouting are concerned is already very well covered in other publications, particularly the *Handbooks* and *Programme Planning in The Scout Troop* by Ron Jefferies: listed below are the additional points which may need to be covered depending on the number of boys with a handicap and the nature of the handicaps. Taken *in toto* they represent the guide lines for a camp primarily for the severely handicapped. In many instances, a boy with a relatively minor handicap can fully participate with little or no adaptations.

Preliminaries

You will already have the basic information about the boy,

his handicap and what general treatment he may need during a Troop or Unit meeting. For camping you will need, for the boy's comfort and enjoyment, certain additional information from the boy's parents and, *via the boy's parents,* from his doctor.

It is suggested that, as well as the usual camp information, etc., the following information be requested:

Bowels: If your son has difficulty sometimes, please give details and say what opening medicines he finds most helpful.

Travelling: If your son is a bad traveller on train or coach, will you please let us know.

Incontinence of urine: Many boys at camp, due to their handicap, are bed-wetters. There is nothing to be ashamed of in this, and it is not a deterrent to their coming to the camp. The Staff will look after them and do the necessary washing, but it is very difficult when we have no previous knowledge of this.

Please answer fully, therefore:

He is incontinent (often
(sometimes
(only at night
(never

Should your boy require frequent changing, *please* send as many spare pants, pyjama trousers, and easily washed shorts or trousers as possible, and see that they are *clearly marked with his name.*

Medicines: All pills must be in a solid container, not a collapsible box. All bottles and containers must be marked with the boy's name, and state time(s) of giving and the dosage.

Treatment: If any special treatment is required inform us in writing on the Camp Permission Form.

Diet: Notify us of any *necessary* diets, so that this can be arranged. If there is difficulty with feeding give us any helpful advice.

Please make a note of any other relevant, useful information. (All such information about your boy will be treated as strictly confidential.)

There should also be a Parents' Consent to Camp form, which is obtainable from Scout Shops Ltd., signed by the boy's parent or guardian and a Camp Medical Certificate signed by the boy's doctor.

Wherever possible take boys with handicaps along for the preliminary site visit. They will be much more likely to be able to point out possible problems themselves than you might imagine by attempting to visualise the site from their point of view.

Preparation

1. Choosing the Site:

It should be flat with easy access. An indoor dormitory should be available where there are boys who are not allowed to sleep under canvas. Baths and/or showers are invaluable particularly for incontinent boys. An indoor hall or marquee is needed for meals and activities (e.g. films, camp fires, etc.) in cold or wet weather. A washing machine in camp or proximity to an all-night launderette is essential.

2. Helpers

Adequate able-bodied help is needed to dress, undress, push chairs, participate in activities, etc. The best age group is 15-18 so that not only physical help but companionship is available (but do not forget that many boys with one type of handicap are capable of – and enjoy – helping those with another type of handicap, and *vice versa).*

Where the camp is primarily for the handicapped, each Patrol should have a Scouter in charge with an assistant, preferably a Venture Scout. There could be non-handicapped Scouts in the Patrol who are fully integrated members of the Patrol: they can be of any age as long as it is remembered that some physically strong boys will be needed for lifting, pushing, etc. Helpers should be shown how to lift a boy with a handicap, how to push chairs over rough ground, etc., and the handicapped boy himself should be encouraged to tell his helper(s) when, where, how and why he needs assistance.

3. Transport

Train, aeroplane or steamer are preferable to coach journeys for travelling to camp. In this country, the train is most convenient but it is expensive and travelling at week-ends can be difficult. Non-stop coach journeys of more than two hours' duration should be avoided, but a long journey split up usually presents little trouble. Aeroplane journeys may not be suitable for all the boys.

In camp some form of suitable transport is essential for emergencies. Separate transport to carry wheelchairs (where there are a number of wheelchair cases) is advisable as coaches can seldom carry many in the luggage compartments.

4. Advance 'Warnings'

(a) In camps primarily for the handicapped it is helpful to have a resident Medical Officer and qualified nursing staff. The nearest doctor and hospital should be advised well in advance of the handicaps of the boys attending camp. If there are any haemophiliacs attending the camp their blood group should be notified to the nearest haemophilia treatment centre.

(b) Notify the local Fire Brigade who will visit the camp and provide portable apparatus. (They may come with an appliance which will provide an interesting and entertaining item on the programme.)

(c) Tell the local Police who can help in many ways, not least of which is traffic control, etc., on local outings.

5. Equipment and kit

(a) A supply of urinal plastic bottles in camp and on outings is essential.

(b) Extra blankets and groundsheets should be taken.

(c) Oilskins are needed for wheelchair cases.

(d) Tents should be high enough to allow helpers to lift and work with the boys, and sufficiently wide to enable easy access with wheelchairs. Boys with handicaps need more room, so fewer can be accommodated in each tent.

(e) additional tents as 'garages' for wheelchairs, and 'stores' for artificial limbs, etc., are advisable.

(f) spare wheelchair parts and an appropriately stocked tool box (with at least one person who can act as 'mechanic').

(g) all personal kit must be clearly marked with its owner's name.

(h) toilet facilities must be suitable. For wheelchair cases, Elsans with hand supports are recommended.

(i) belts are required to strap in those in wheelchairs.

(j) specially designed eating and drinking aids for the severely handicapped should be taken where necessary.

6. Menu

(a) Any special diets must be considered beforehand (the necessary information should be forthcoming on the Camp Permission Certificate).

In Camp

1. Cooking

(a) Can be done either centrally or by Patrols. It will generally be found that central cooking is the most practical, but Patrol cooking should be undertaken for some of the meals during camp.

(b) Altar type fires are preferable for all concerned, particularly those in wheelchairs, but heat shields must be provided to guard against paralysed limbs becoming scorched.

2. Programme

(a) No variation in general programme for camp is necessary.

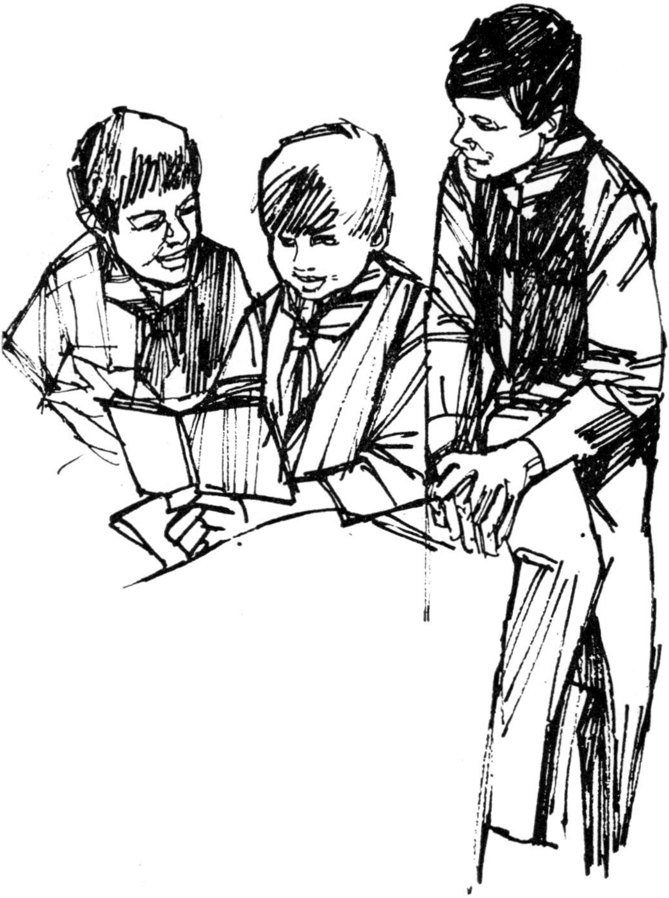

(b) Inspection of site and kit should be in accord with camping standards, but as far as the individual is concerned the boy should be inspected for cleanliness but should not be expected to get into uniform where it is a long and tedious operation for both the boy with the handicap and his helper. Uniform should be worn only for travelling to and from camp and for outings to town (but not on expeditions).
(c) Outings and visits – places should be visited beforehand to check such details as access, toilet facilities, etc.

3. Welfare

(a) Hygiene is always of great importance at any Scout camp, but is of *paramount* importance where boys with handicaps are concerned as many are more susceptible to infection or contracting illnesses.
(b) One Scouter and one Venture Scout should be on duty all the time, and take watches throughout the night. This will not only give the boys an assurance that there is someone *awake* who can help them if neccesary, but will also ensure that there is someone to attend to those who need turning regularly (e.g. those with muscular dystrophy).

The Intellectually Handicapped

General

What follows applies particularly to the educationally handicapped who are members of Extension Groups, but the information should also be of use to those Leaders who have boys in their Sections who have some degree of intellectual handicap. Chapter 5 described, in general terms, the nature of intellectual handicaps.

Outdoor Activities

Scouting encourages independent thought and action in educationally handicapped children to equip them for the world when they leave school. This striving towards independence in the individual child through Scout activities also arouses in the boy the realisation of the value of the co-operation of the group, no matter how small, for the benefit and sometimes for the personal safety of each member of the group.

Training for outdoor activities will, of course, need to be 'broken down' into a number of very simple stages, each of which needs to be understood. The correct sequence of these stages needs to be remembered, not by theoretical talks and instruction, but by constant practical repetition 'on the ground'.

A member of the staff of a Special School writes: 'Scout

activities frequently produce the exact situation to make our slow learners think independently. *Situations* arise which have to be assessed, a *judgement* has to be maae on that assessment, a *decision* has to be made on how to act on that judgement, and lastly the *action* has to be effected.

'It is quite amazing to watch a slow learner rock climbing and then traversing to the ground. He has to do numerous logical actions in a particular order: should he make one incorrectly or in the incorrect order, then he would be in some personal danger. Of course, in the initial stages life-lines are used. This exercise in remembered logical sequence is tremendous training for the children, and the resultant gaining of individual self-confidence and the satisfaction of doing a job well, is invaluable.

'Scouting can help to create an industrious environment free from petty squabbles, irritations and strife. Children are naturally curious. Colour and movement attract their eye. They want to explore. They constantly ask the great questions of "How?" and "Why?" and they want their questions answered. Scouting helps the boys to have their curiosity broadened, their interests broadened and their enthusiasms encouraged. These activities can become part of the wholesome education of these children. With guidance, the slow learner will become very much aware of the world around him.

'The children's capabilities must be realised, and the training methods applicable to their low level of attainment. In the progressive stages of Scouting a wide variety of interests can be pursued but there is a limit to the slow learner's accomplishment. Practical activities are the most beneficial. Children at this school regularly take part in pioneering, swimming, sailing, athletics, canoeing, camping, expedition training, first aid and rock climbing. Because many slow learners are physically fit, no modification in the standard is required.'

Camping

1. *SITE:* Because slow learners do tend to show themselves up in a poor light, even though they are very willing to 'have a go', the site should be relatively secluded and not too much on show to other Scouts or the general public.

2. *PRACTICAL CONSIDERATIONS:* Many slow learners are bedwetters or soil themselves. When accepted as 'a fact of life' by the Leaders, the boys are much less likely to be embarrassed with the resultant relieving of emotional stress and the reduction of the likelihood of this happening. The boys should have plastic sheets or bed covers, and bed

sheets and blankets should be used rather than sleeping bags. A good stock of spare sheets is necessary. If a washing machine is not available at the site, it is advisable to be relatively close to an all-night launderette.

3. Programme

(a) needs to be very full with plenty of variety.

(b) visits, hikes, etc., should be undertaken as a collective Troop effort.

4. The Patrol System

(a) The Patrol system and cooking by Patrols should be limited to week-end camps and then only when at least one of the adult staff is available to attend each Patrol in an advisory capacity.

(b) For camps of longer duration than a week-end, central cooking is more advantageous, and the Patrol system used for all other activities.

Troops of slow learners have reached the top three or four in County Camping Competitions.

CHAPTER 9

Uniform

1. The Cub Scout's, Scout's or Venture Scout's uniform is his visible identification with the Scout Movement. The young man with a handicap is particularly proud of his uniform as it is exactly the same uniform as all the other Cub Scouts, Scouts or Venture Scouts wear. This outward sign of his acceptance by his fellows, and of his sense of belonging, can be a powerful factor in promoting his self-respect and confidence in himself.

2. Because of the nature of a boy's physical structure, it will sometimes be necessary to make alterations to the uniform to allow for various deformities and to ensure the boy is comfortable when wearing his uniform, and can more easily get into and out of the uniform himself. All alterations are designed to be as inconspicuous as possible and to minimise the disfigurement or disability.

3. The psychological value of a boy with a handicap having a *new* uniform, even if it has to be altered, far outweighs economic considerations. No boy with a handicap should have a secondhand uniform, whether or not it has to be altered. Parents should be given financial help by a loan or grant from Group, District or County funds.

4. In most instances, adaptations are relatively simple and can be done by anyone skilful with a needle; only occasionally will more expert help be needed. The following suggestions are primarily intended for Leaders to pass on to parents. Leaders could discuss the matter with the parents (or the Matron of a Special Boarding School) *before* the uniform is purchased so that, if necessary, the size of a particular part of the uniform can allow for alterations.

5. *SPECIAL MATERIALS* mentioned in this chapter:

'Velcro' touch and close fastener – Selectus Ltd., Biddulph, Stoke-on-Trent, and most drapers.

'Staflex' Adhesive, iron-on interfacing – McCulloch and Wallis Ltd., 25/26 Dering Street, London, W.1. and some drapers.

'Latafoam' patches – Latafoam Ltd., 199 High Holborn, London, W.C.2.

Foam laminate – Nottingham Handcraft Co., Melton Road, Nottingham, and most drapers.

Kiwi Stretch-laces and So-Esi Laces (Radiol Chemicals) – most shoe shops and shoe-repairers.

Headgear

General:

Never secure headgear with elastic under the chin.

Cub Scout Cap

1. Where a boy has difficulty in keeping his cap on, insert a band of rubberised tape (obtainable from most drapers) round the 'rim' behind the peak.
2. If a Cub's head is too large for the largest sized Cub cap or his head is mis-shaped, it may be better to discourage him from wearing any headgear as it could accentuate his deformity.

Scout/Venture Scout Beret

1. The leather band will usually hold the beret in position.
2. If a Scout's head is large, the leather can be removed, and replaced by black elastic which should be at least ¾in. wide to prevent it 'cutting' the skin.

Jerseys and Shirts

Cub Scout Jerseys and T-shirts

1. Where crutches are used jerseys and T-shirts may require reinforcing under the arms.
2. Where a boy is confined to a wheelchair the jersey may need reinforcing at the elbow and under the forearm.

Scout/Venture Scout Shirts

1. *SIZE.* Where a boy uses his arms to propel a wheelchair or for crutch walking, he may need a shirt slightly larger than his normal size, to give breadth across the shoulders. Untucking during such exercise can be avoided by lengthening the shirt by 2in. or 3in.
2. *FASTENINGS* are one of the greatest obstacles to a boy being able to dress and undress himself.

On the shirt front *buttons* may be removed and be re-attached on top of the buttonhole. Then do one of the following:

(a) Stitch one 1in. square of *'Velcro'* to the place where each button was, and another 1in. square of 'Velcro' behind each buttonhole. When pressed together the 'Velcro' squares adhere to one another, and pull apart easily for undressing.
(b) attach *press-studs* instead of 'Velcro'. These are more difficult to do up than 'Velcro', but are easier than buttons.
(c) use a zip-fastener, which should preferably be open-ended and reach from the top button to 3in. from the bottom

of the shirt. Attach a ring or tab to the puller to enable the wearer to use the zip easily. Where a boy has difficulty in getting the open ends of the zip together, sew up the bottom 6in. of the shirt flaps and use a closed-end zip.
At *the cuffs* buttons can be attached to thin elastic (see diagram 1) or a loop of elastic can be sewn between the cuff ends and the button attached to the top of the button-hole.

Diagram 1

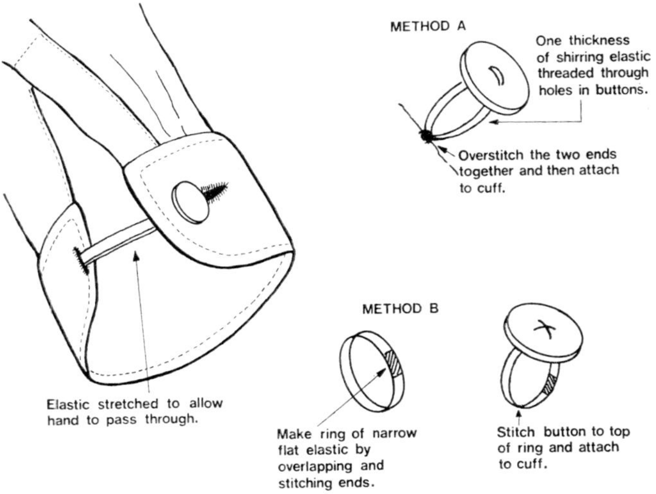

3. *REINFORCEMENT* or *EASING* may be necessary at certain points of wear or strain (e.g. under arms, particularly if crutches are used).
Either: (a) Attach 'Staflex' Adhesive iron-on interfacing to areas requiring extra strength, or
(b) double machine along seams, or
(c) Machine or stitch 3/4in. to 1in. tape along the back of any seam under strain (see diagram 2) or
(d) Insert gussets at points of strain. Open a seam near the place where more fullness is needed, and insert a strip of similar material (see diagram 3).

Diagram 2

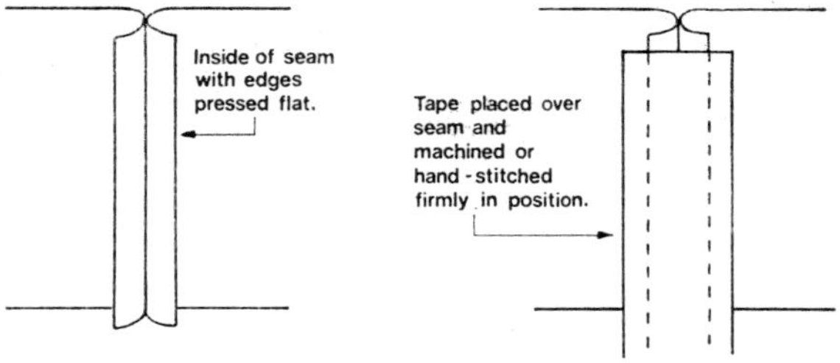

4. *SLEEVE ADAPTATION* (e.g. if arms are of unequal length) is best done at the elbow crease. To shorten, take up a tuck: to lengthen insert a piece of similar material.

Scout/Venture Scout Trousers

A waistband can be constricting when boys have to sit in wheelchairs for long periods. A size larger than usual should be more comfortable and will also help to prevent the trousers 'dragging' arround the thighs if the boy slides in the chair: it often makes 'toiletting' easier. Any 'over fullness' at the waist can be corrected by inserting elastic through the waistband at the back.

Diagram 3

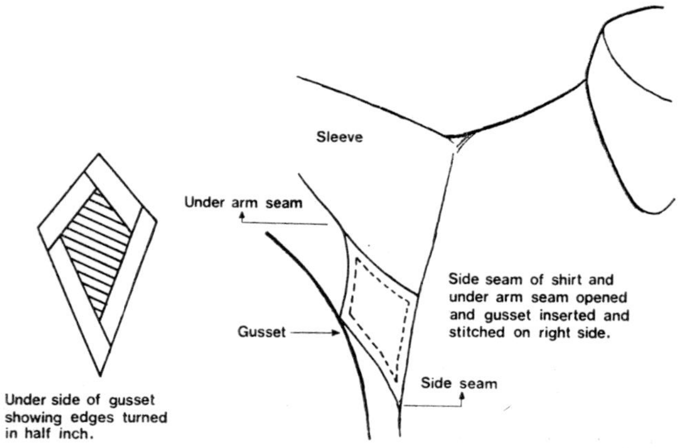

If, despite lengthening, the shirt still tends to pull out, sew a strip of rubberised petersham on to the trouser waistband. Where trouser legs need adjustment, turn up at the bottom. Other adaptations which may be necessary or useful:

1. *FASTENINGS*

(a) Substitute *'Velcro'* for the usual *waistband* fastening.

(b) Attach one *tab* or *loop* to the puller of the zip *fly-front fastener* and another tab to the bottom of the zip to give the boy an anchor when pulling. Arrange the bottom tab to tuck out of sight behind the fly fold when the zip is closed (see diagram 4).

Diagram 4

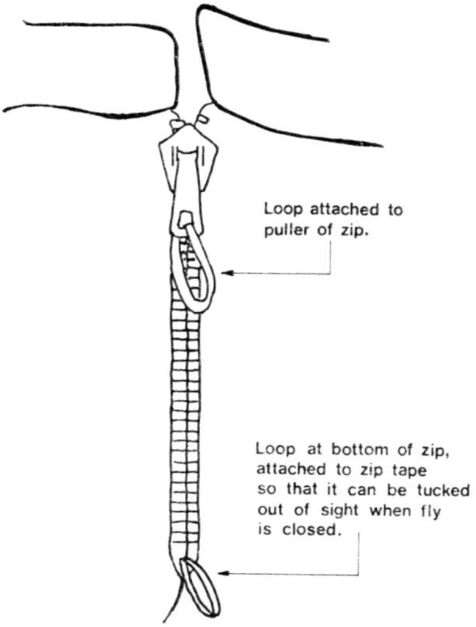

(c) An upside down zip to open the fly from the bottom may be useful where arm movement is restricted by stiffness of shoulders or elbows. As the waistband will be permanently closed, it will need to be elasticated. The back seam may have to be opened and a gusset inserted (see diagram 5), OR one or both side seams can be open for about 9in. and zips or *'Velcro'* inserted.

2. *REINFORCEMENT* at points of strain or pressure, particularly if callipers are worn. Use one of the following:

(a) iron-on facing material.

(b) a strong, smooth material (e.g. nylon). Patches can be attached with special fabric glue which is washable.

(c) special 'Latafoam' patches.

OR: line the trousers completely with strong nylon. This has

Diagram 5

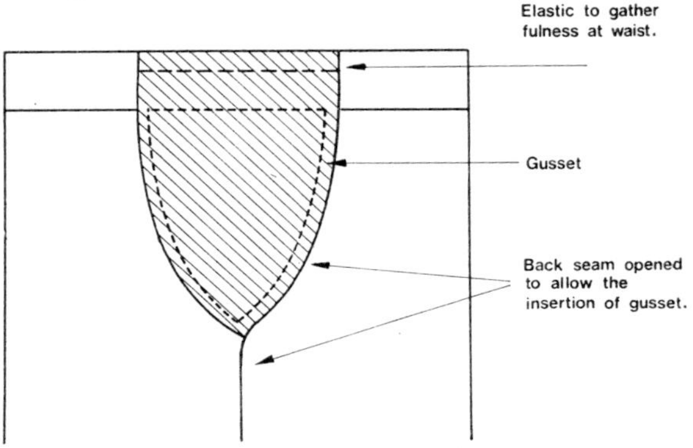

the additional advantage of increasing warmth and the trousers will slip on more easily.

3. *OPENINGS*

Many Scouts with handicaps, particularly those with stiff ankles or those wearing callipers, need an opening in the seam at the lower part of each leg. Inner or outer seams may be opened and *'Velcro'* or zips inserted. With *'Velcro'* a strip of facing material should be stitched to one side of the opened seam to form a backing on which the *'Velcro'* can be machined. (See diagram 6.)

Diagram 6

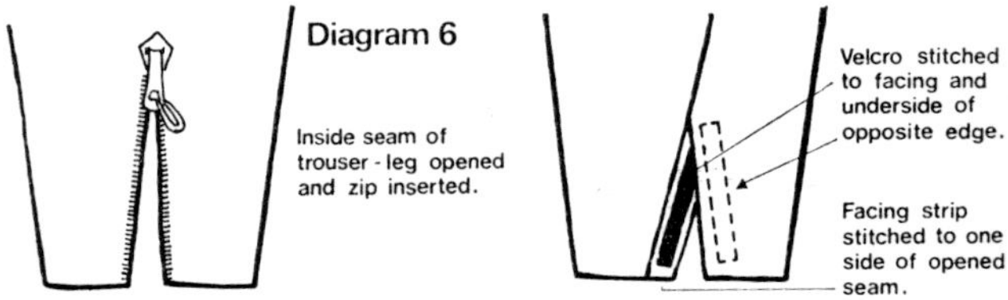

Shorts (Cub Scouts)

Adaptations, where necessary, can be carried out as for trousers.

Where a handicap to the lower limbs requires warmth or protection, trousers should be worn, preferably of a similar colour and material to the shorts worn by others in the Pack.

Outer Garment

(a) *Cuff* fastenings may require adaptation (as for shirt).
(b) *Loops* or *tabs* may be needed on the *zip* (as for trousers).
(c) If a boy finds the initial linking at the bottom of the zip

impossible, it can be replaced with toggles (see diagram 7).

Diagram 7

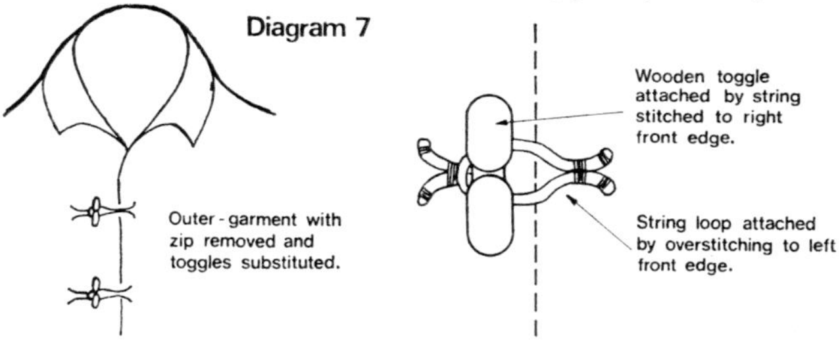

(d) A lining of *foam laminate* gives additional warmth without weight: a larger size garment than usual will be needed.

Belts

The standard fastening is fairly easy to manipulate. Magnetic fastenings can be obtained, and a shoe repairer can do the adaptation.

Shoes

Although some boys wear elasticated shoes, many prefer lace-up ones, and they may have difficulty in putting them on and tying the laces, either because they cannot reach their feet easily, or because they lack manual dexterity or co-ordination.

EITHER: Replace laces with 1/4in. black or brown elastic. The bow once tied, can be stitched to keep it fastened. The elastic stretches sufficiently for the foot to be inserted in the shoe without untying the laces.

OR: buy 'stretch-laces.'

(a) A shoe-lace can be tied with one hand (see diagram 8).

Diagram 8

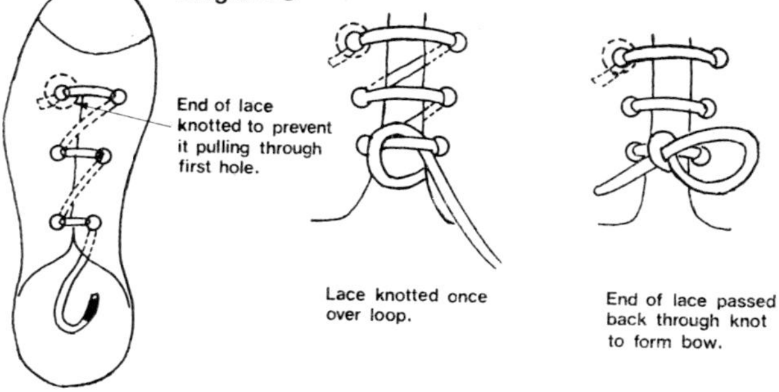

(b) If a boy finds difficulty in reaching his feet, try a long-handled shoehorn which can be bought or made by fixing a rod to an ordinary shoehorn with screws.

Diagram 9

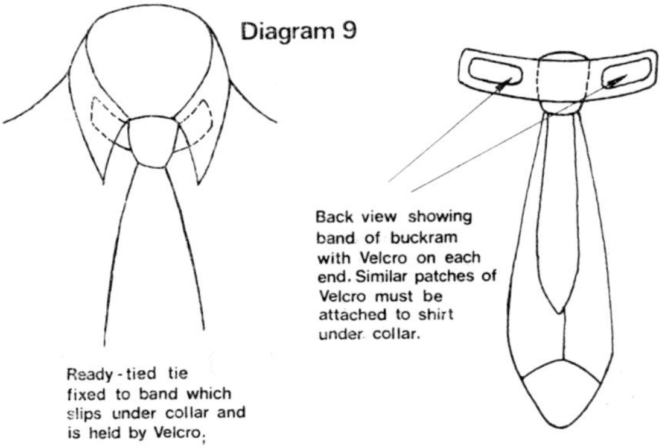

(c) Laces can be replaced with a zip (put in by a shoe repairer) which can be opened and closed with a hooked stick.

Scarves

Scarves present little difficulty, but a *woggle* may, particularly if a boy has only one good hand. Make a woggle which will wrap around the scarf, fastening with a press-stud or *'Velcro'*.

Ties

For those boys who cannot tie a tie, make a *ready knotted* tie stitched either to elastic or to a band, which can be fixed under the collar with 'Velcro' (see diagram 9).

APPENDIX I

Amending Badge Requirements

As stated previously the responsibility for deciding whether a Badge requirement needs to be amended and what the amendments are to be is that of the Section Leader. He can, of course, seek the advice and help of the District or County Extension Activities Adviser. The suggestions which follow are intended only as guide-lines.

When devising equivalent requirements, equal challenge and the need for comparable effort should be considered as for the existing ones. Also, they should meet the same purpose with a similar expectancy of success.

Cub Scouts

Bronze Arrow

Feats of Skill

The first requirement is designed to develop the co-ordination of the senses.

(a) A boy with gross unco-ordination of the arms and eyes could be encouraged to improve his co-ordination by manipulating and handling, for example, in the construction of a simple Airfix model.

(b) The physically handicapped, without the use of their hands might kick a ball to another boy standing 16ft. (5 metres) away, or into a narrow-mouthed 'goal'. With only the limited use of hands, a 'table' ball game offers possibilities.

(c) The visually handicapped could use a 'blimp' ball or a bell ball.

The second requirement necessitates physical activity.

(a) The physically handicapped who has use of his hands but is in a wheelchair could demonstrate his skill in manoeuvring his wheel chair between obstacles, etc. If this is impossible, the scope of another bronze arrow requirement could be extended (e.g. discovering nature) or a new requirement substituted (e.g. making a collection).

Handcraft

The physically handicapped, if unable to use his hands,

could attempt to paint a picture holding the brush in his mouth or between his toes.

Knotting

If it is not possible to tie knots, the boy could direct another boy on how to do it.

Silver Arrow

Feats of Skill

If both swimming and the alternative requirements are impossible, a boy could learn more about the safety rules for the requirements, or choose a sport and know the basic rules of the game (e.g. so he could umpire or referee Pack soccer, cricket, rounders and such like games).

Discovering Nature

The blind could be encouraged to develop their knowledge of nature with their other senses, e.g. *touch:* tree bark; *smell:* identifying flowers, vegetables or herbs; *hearing:* bird calls; *taste:* fruit.

Safety

The water safety rules should be known as they provide useful information to pass on to others.

Service

For using the telephone – the deaf could use a telephone with a light instead of a bell, be encouraged to speak and to use simple answering sentences. If no speech, encourage the use of the telephone directory (including the yellow pages) as an aid in the home and the Dialling Code book. The message for the educationally handicapped will need to be very simple. A substitute requirement could be to understand the units of currency.

Out-of-doors

A 'Gaz' stove can be used instead of a wood-fire.

Knotting

Similar to Bronze suggestion.

Gold Arrow

Health

Instead of *making* a First Aid Kit the Cub Scout could *choose* the contents of the kit. He could direct another Cub Scout to tie a sling and to deal with a sprained ankle.

Feats of Skill

Similar to Silver suggestion, which could be developed further.

Exploring

The blind could learn how to read an embossed map or how to use a Braille compass.

Discovering Nature

For the physically handicapped without the use of hands a tape recording could be substituted for a log or a collection.

Knotting

Similar to Bronze suggestion.

Scouts

The Scout Standard

Looking After Yourself

Encourage boys to meet the requirements but, if necessary, substitute 'day out' for 'camp'. What is important is that the boy should do something different, getting away from four walls, away from home.

Getting About

The blind can use an embossed map and a braille compass. For the hike, the physically handicapped and the educationally handicapped could use a portable tape recorder on the journey. A Scout in a wheelchair could go with his Patrol and the journey's length be 5 kms (3 miles).

Scouting Skills

Using a knife and an axe: the blind and physically handicapped should use a saw instead.
Weather: the blind could develop a sense of sounds in relation to the weather.

The Advanced Scout Standard

Self Reliance

Swimming: Show an ability to move in the water. The exact distance should be varied depending on the ability of the Scout concerned, and should be a challenge for him. There may be cases where this requirement cannot be met, and a suitable alternative, designed for the Scout concerned to show he has an ability to follow instructions, be substituted.
Menu and cooking: Tell another Scout how to cook. Go on a shopping expedition to cover a two-man week-end camp.

Adventure

The journey: the length of the journey may need to be reduced. A tape recording about the journey could be substituted for the brief written account.
Place of interest or day out: Private transport can be used but the Scout with a handicap should always be accompanied by another Scout or Scouts.

Scoutcraft

Pioneering: it is important that the physically handicapped or blind should take an *active* part in the Patrol project and not just watch.
Backwoods meal or making a bivouac: it may be necessary to omit this in certain circumstances.
Visit: this could be a Patrol, rather than an individual project, where disabling circumstances necessitate.
Passing a Pursuit Badge: where necessary, an Interest Badge could be substituted.

APPENDIX II

Some Useful Addresses

The National Kidney Research Fund, 54 Paddington Street, London, W1M 3RQ.
Renal Unit, Dulwich Hospital, East Dulwich Grove, London, S.E.22.
Royal National Institute for the Deaf, 105 Gower Street, London, W.C.1.
The National Deaf Children's Society, 31 Gloucester Place, London, W1H 4EA.
British Migraine Association, 6 Bryanstone Road, Bournemouth, Hants.
The Spastics Society, 12 Park Crescent, London, W1N 4EQ.
The Chest and Heart Association, Tavistock House North, Tavistock Square, London, W.C.1.
The Haemophilia Society, P.O. Box 9, 16 Trinity Street, London, S.E.1.
National Elfrida Rathbone Society, Toynbee Hall, 28 Commercial Street, London, E.1.
National Society for Mentally Handicapped Children, 86 Newman Street, London, W1P 4AR.
National Association for Mental Health, 39 Queen Anne Street, London, W.1.
National Fund for Research into Crippling Diseases, Vincent House, Vincent Square, London, S.W.1.
PHAB, National Association for Youth Clubs, 30 Devonshire Street, London, W1N 2AP.
Central Council for the Disabled, 34 Eccleston Square, London, S.W.1.
Invalid Children's Aid Association, 126 Buckingham Palace Road, London, S.W.1.

Shaftesbury Society, 112 Regency Street, London, S.W.1.
British Epilepsy Association, 3-6 Alfred Place, London, W.C.1.
Association for Spina Bifida and Hydrocephalus, 112 City Road, London, EC1V 2ND.
British Diabetic Association, 3-6 Alfred Place, London, W.C.1.
The Multiple Sclerosis Society, 4 Tachbrook Street, London, S.W.1.
National Society for Autistic Children, 1a Golders Green Road, London, N.W.11.
The British Polio Fellowship, Clifton House, Euston Road, London, N.W.1.
Muscular Dystrophy Group of Great Britain, 26 Borough High Street, London, S.E.1.
Royal National Institute for the Blind, 224 Great Portland Street, London, W1N 6AA.
The Guide Dogs for the Blind Association, Clifton House, 83-89 Uxbridge Road, Ealing, London, W.5.
Migraine Trust, 23 Queen Square, London, W.C.1.
The Cystic Fibrosis Research Trust, 5 Blyth Road, Bromley, Kent, DR1 3RS.
The National Federation of Gateway Clubs, 86 Newman Street, London, W1P 4AR.

Acknowledgements

The Scout Association extends its sincere thanks to all those individuals, Societies and Organisations that have assisted in the compilation of this book, and in particular:

Past (ø) and Present (*) members of the National Extension Activities Board:

- * **J. A. Allen,** Assistant Director of Leader Training, Gilwell Park.
- * **A. Andrews,** District Extension Adviser, Medvale, Manchester.
- * **S. P. Ansell,** County Commissioner, West Denbighshire.
- ø **G. V. H. Baerlein,** Assistant Director of Leader Training, Gilwell Park.
- ø **Miss B. Baker,** Training Secretary, The Girl Guides Association.
- ***R. B. Barnes,** B.Sc., Assistant County Commissioner (Extension Activities), Essex.
- ø **A. Bolton,** Field Commissioner and past Secretary, National Extension Activities Board.
- ø **Miss B. E. G. Collins,** formerly Assistant County Commissioner (Extension Activities), Oxfordshire.
- * **H. J. G. Collis,** T.D., M.A., Chief Commissioner, Programme and Training.

* **B. V. Dightam,** C.Eng., District Commissioner, North Leeds, and Assistant Leader Trainer.

* **Dr. S. N. Donaldson,** M.D., D.P.H., Northern Ireland Headquarters Adviser, Extension Activities.

* **Mrs. G. A. Drew,** Assistant Headquarters Commissioner for Extension Activities.

A. T. S. Edwards, Physical Education Adviser, The Spastics Society.

ø **G. S. Dunn,** Home Office Inspector.

ø **J. Fish,** H.M.I., Department of Education and Science.

ø **R. C. Gover,** Assistant County Commissioner (Extension Activities), Bristol.

ø **D. G. Griffiths,** Assistant County Commissioner (Extension Activities), Shropshire.

* **A. C. Hammond,** Headquarters Commissioner for Extension Activities.

ø **E. W. Hayden,** Executive Commissioner (Administration) and Secretary.

ø **A. W. Hurll,** C.V.O., C.B.E., formerly Chief Executive Commissioner.

* **J. B. Huskins,** M.A., Director of Leader Training, Gilwell Park.

* **A. V. Kemp,** Dip. Ed., Executive Commissioner, Programme and Training.

* **Dr. B. Kiernander,** M.B., M.R.C.P., D.M.R.E., D.Phys.Med., Director of Physical Medicine, Hospital for Sick Children, Great Ormond Street, London.

A. T. Mellowship, F.I.B.S.T., Renal Unit, Dulwich Hospital.

* **T. A. Morris,** Assistant Scout Leader, 225th North London.

ø **A. M. Munday,** H.M.I., E.R.D., Department of Education and Science.

ø **J. N. Pryce,** J.P., B.A., Assistant County Commissioner for Scouts, North West Lancashire.

ø **L. A. Robinson,** O.B.E., C.Eng., Chairman, World Extension Scouting Sub-Committee.

* **Mrs. W. M. Robinson,** Extension Adviser, The Girl Guides Association.

ø **M. Sloane,** Field Commissioner and past Secretary, National Extension Activities Board.

* **Mrs. E. Smith,** District Extension Adviser, Bletchley & Wolverton.

* **K. H. Stevens,** M.I.M., Chief Executive Commissioner.

* **J. Sutton-Pratt,** Secretary, National Extension Activities Board.

Mrs. M. Wallis, S.R.N., former member of Service Team, County of London.

* **L. B. Watson,** Scottish Headquarters Adviser, Extension Activities.
D. L. Webb, Assistant County Commissioner (Extension Activities), Wiltshire.
ø **Lady Jean Wemyss,** formerly Extension Adviser, The Girl Guides Association.
* **R. J. Wiltshire,** Assistant County Commissioner (Extension Activities), Somerset.
ø **T. Wylie,** B.A., Assistant Director of Leader Training, Gilwell Park.
The Association for Spina Bifida and Hydrocephalus.
British Diabetic Association.
British Migraine Association.
British Polio Fellowship.
Burton Hill House School for Physically Handicapped Children.
The Chest and Heart Association.
The Department of Education and Science.
Department of Physical Medicine, Hospital for Sick Children, Great Ormond Street, London.
Epilepsy Information Unit of the British Epilepsy Association
The Haemophilia Society.
Medical Research Council Unit for Physical Aids for the Disabled.
Muscular Dystrophy Group of Great Britain.
National Association for Mental Health.
National Elfrida Rathbone Society.
The National Deaf Children's Society.
National Society for Autistic Children.
National Society for Mentally Handicapped Children.
Royal National Institute for the Blind.
Royal National Institute for the Deaf.

We are able to publish this book at the subsidised cover price through generous help received from the **Treloar Handicapped Scouts Fund.**

Index

We have listed the Physical and Invisible Handicaps covered in Chapters 4 and 5 in alphabetical order for easy reference.

ALSO BY DAVID CAVANAGH

The Middleman, 2003

Pythia: A Dramatic Poem, 1989

Ethic = Visceral, 1987